YOGA FOR BEGINNERS

YOGA MAGIC!

Best Gentle Yoga Poses to Relieve Stress, Improve Relaxation, and Have A Satisfying Stretch

SONIA BYRD

Table of Contents

PART I

Your Restorative Practice

Restorative Yoga is a calming practice. A practice that many of us need daily.

This specific type of yoga helps to release tension, anxiety and stress that stems from busy daily activities, traumatic circumstance or life-changing events. Restorative yoga typically utilizes props including blankets, bolsters, blocks, aromatherapy, etc. Props in restorative yoga assist with body alignment, relaxation and weight balance. They can also aide in alleviating pressure in certain areas of the body while practicing asanas.

Most of us are aware of the popular yoga classes that incorporate constant movement and active poses. Restorative yoga, however, utilizes the poses that allow your body to slowly stretch in to a relaxed state. Breathing techniques and meditation are incorporated into each pose prompting the body to slow down and enter a mode of stillness. These restorative poses and techniques ease symptoms related to anxiety, depression, stress, pain and trauma-related injuries.

The main ingredient in restorative yoga is time and patience. Each pose is held for a longer period of time allowing the body to enter into a state of mind-body unification. Holding the poses for a longer period of time also provides a deeper stretch, "stretching to the bone," as some would explain.

Daily life can send us reeling through a multitude of emotions. Simply going to the grocery store can ingnite a high level of stress. Unexpected, life-altering events may bring about intense changes affecting the way we react to certain situations. The way we handle stressful situations can cause the physical body to remain tense with no sign of relief. The human body is capable of leading a very active life. We must take the time to give our minds and our bodies a break. If we do not, our immune system might deteriorate, and our minds will fade.

So, when do we slow down?

More importantly, how do we slow down? Once that roller coaster called life starts chugging away, most of us don't know how to stop, or how to slow down. We need some kind of assistance or daily practice that will help us to decompress. We must stop running ourselves into the ground.

Learning how to recognize a quiet moment, a peaceful place, the sound of silence – We all long for each of those opportunities, but refuse to stop and realize that they are most likely right in front of our faces. Stillness is very important. And, the older we get, the harder it is to return to that state of stillness.

Generally speaking, yoga is defined as the unification of the mind and body. It is the practice of harmonizing the physical body with the spiritual body and returning to a conscious state of stillness and mindfulness.

When practicing the restorative method of yoga, time is a very important aspect. In restorative yoga, you will hold the asanas for 3-5x longer than in other yoga practices. Typically, in one restorative yoga session, you may only complete 3-5 poses. As opposed to an active yoga session, you may flow continuously through 10-20 poses.

Some examples of restorative yoga poses are Child's pose, Corpse pose, Legs-Up-The-Wall pose, etc. During each pose, you can incorporate very specific breathing techniques and meditation methods. Holding the poses for a longer period of time also allows you to adjust your body for proper alignment and balance.

Let's face it, we are all uniquely built. Not one of us is the same, physically, emotionally or mentally. Therefore, we must adjust our yoga practice to fit our own personal needs.

There are many ways to create your own unique restorative yoga practice.

Yoga is for Everyone

First of all, let's get one thing straight. You do not have to be perfect to practice any type of yoga. Yoga is a balancing of the mind and the body. We all have very unique body types. No one is made the same. Your yoga practice is exactly just that - a practice tailored to fit the needs of your mind and your body.

You may feel

like you are overweight, too tall, too short, not flexible, too skinny, etc. Try to let go of whatever inhibitions may be keeping you from jumping into your first routine. Many people immediately associate the word yoga with headstands and pretzel poses. While those advanced activities are certainly a piece of the yoga puzzle, they do not define yoga.

For example, let's say you have had a really rough day at the office, or with the kiddos. Maybe you are dealing with a loss in the family or financial struggles. Maybe your day, week, month or year just hasn't gone as planned. If you know the basics of yoga and how to practice on your own, you just may be able to ease that anxiety or calm the stress that comes during those difficult times.

But, hey! Maybe you are having a great day, week, month or year. That sounds wonderful, doesn't it? Then let your yoga practice serve that cherry on top. Learning the simple art of taking breaths throughout your day and mastering the act of sitting still could totally change your life.

There's nothing wrong with feeling shy at first when it comes to deciding to start your own yoga practice. But, remember, you are important and need to be healthy and happy. Taking that first step toward the local yoga studio or even just setting up a yoga mat at home could be one of the best steps of your life!

A Restorative Practice at Home

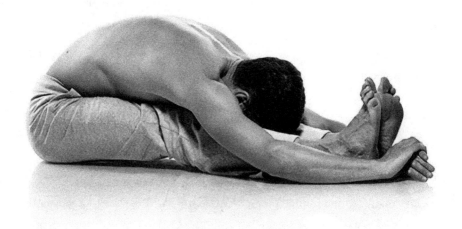

Restorative Yoga can absolutely be practiced at home.

Gyms and studios are fabulous practice areas as well. But, there may be days where you can't make it out of the house. Or, your schedule isn't permitting a quick run to the gym. Sometimes yoga studios have to reorganize their classes and you usual time slot isn't available anymore.

That's ok!

Let's create our own home studio for those days.

Follow these simple steps to begin setting up your own home practice.

1. Find a Quiet Spot - Find a space in your home away from loud noises and people. That space may be in a quiet room, in the backyard, or any peaceful spot that you choose.

2. Set the Mood - Once you have found the perfect space, dim the lights, lower the shades and turn down any loud sounds. If you enjoy a favorite scent, turn on

an oil diffuser, light a candle, or burn incense.

3. Create Space - Yoga requires space. Once your yoga mat is situated, make sure to move any objects that may get in the way of your arms and legs.

4. Be Patient - Practicing yoga at home is very different than practicing in a studio. There may be times when you have to check on the kids, answer the door, check the oven, etc. That's ok. Simply deciding to begin yoga is a huge step in the right direction.

Breathing Techniques

Each yoga pose should include a breathing pattern, or breathing technique if you will. There are many types of breathing patterns to follow. It is perfectly acceptable to create a breathing pace that works best for your practice.

Let's face it, we all lack the proper amount of oxygen. We readily give in to the ease of shallow breathing throughout our busy day, and we forget to take in those absolutely necessary deep breaths.

The practice of breathing in yoga is called Pranayama.

If yoga does nothing other than prompt us to breath for an hour, then so be it. In fact, if you are a beginner yoga student, simply just learning how to breath may be the extent of your first few classes. Enjoy it, because the hard poses come next!

Practicing how to breath seems like a simple task. Just wait though. This involuntary act of breathing that we so recklessly abandon too much in a day may give you that energy boost you've been looking for. And, guess what? You can practice breathing anywhere!

So, let's breath.

Pursed Lip Breathing

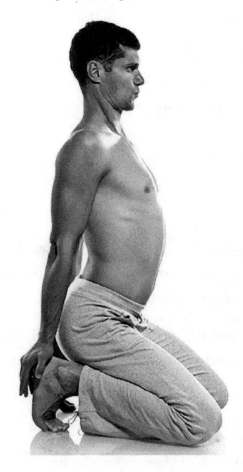

1. Sit quietly and relax your neck and shoulders. Place your arms beside your body and let your hands lay on your lap or mat.

2. Inhale through your nose and hold for two counts.

3. Purse your lips as if you were drinking through a straw.

4. Gently blow your entire breath out through your lips until your abdomen releases completely.

Diaphragm Breathing

1. Lie on your back in a quiet space. You can bend your knees for comfort or simply rest both legs on the floor.

2. Place one hand on your chest and the other hand on your stomach.

3. Inhale through your nose allowing your belly to extend.

4. Exhale through your pursed lips, feeling your belly empty all of its air, releasing down into your spine.

Lion's Breathing

1. Sit comfortably in a quiet space with legs crossed and hands placed on both knees.

2. Inhale through your nose letting your chest expand. Lower both shoulders.

3. Open your mouth wide and exhale making the "Ha" sound until you've expended all of the air in your belly.

Alternate Nostril Breathing

1. Begin in a seated position

2. Lift your hand to your nose. Press your pointer and middle finger down against your palm and release the index and pinky fingers toward the sky.

3. Press your thumb against your right nostril. Closing the airway.

4. Inhale through your left nostril.

5. Release the thumb and exhale through your right nostril.

6. Repeat on the other side.

Coherent Breathing

1. Find a comfortable seated position

2. Inhale for 5 counts.

3. Exhale for 5 counts.

Any one of these breathing techniques can be performed during your restorative yoga practice. The beauty behind the art of breathing is that it can be done anywhere, preferably in a quiet and calm space.

There are, however, many times during the day where you are not able to find a quiet space. Let's say you begin to feel anxious during an important business meeting. You could quietly begin the "Coherent Breathing" technique without causing a scene.

Not only can you practice these breathing steps during a restorative yoga session, but you can also apply them in everyday situations.

Meditation Methods

Meditatiion in an intergral piece to every type of yoga practice. In fact, meditation should be an important part of each person's daily routine. There is no one way to meditate. Personal meditation practices are based each person's unique character, specific surroundings and life experiences.

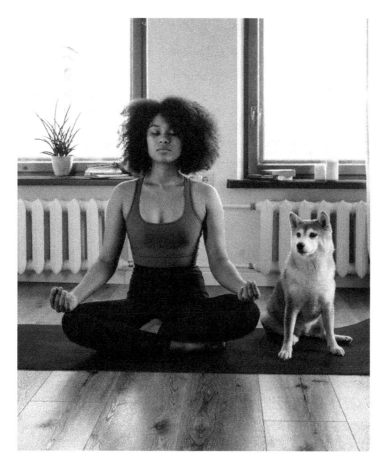

There are hundreds of meditation techniques spanning many different cultures, religions and spiritual practices. Choosing a meditation method that is right for you may take time. It is important to find the right space – space where you feel comfortable enough to be yourself.

Meditation is your personal piece of art. Your thoughts during meditation are your own and belong to no one else. It is a time for you to be honest with yourself. This is your space to approach the places in your mind that are typically suppressed in real life.

There are two types of meditation – guided and unguided.

Guided meditation is exactly as it sounds. A teacher helps to guide you through the steps of a particular meditation practice. The teacher explains how the mind operates, walks you through step-by-step and assists in implementing the meditation into your daily life.

Unguided meditation simply involves one person – You. This method of meditation allows you to decide exactly where, when and how you want to practice. You are the teacher when it comes to an unguided meditation practice.

Simply put, meditation teaches focus. Our day-to-day lives are constantly filled with messages, ads, phone calls, texts, requests, deadlines, etc. Our brain never gets a moment to itself. Meditation is the art of finally stopping all the ruckus in your head and giving your personal thoughts some much needed attention.

As we continue to deal with all of these distractions, our mind becomes adept to wandering. We never get the chance to complete our thoughts. We are constantly distracted.

Meditation teaches us how to recognize when our mind begins to wander away from the initial thought. As you practice mindfulness in meditation, you learn how to bring your thoughts back to consciousness and awareness.

In restorative yoga, meditation can be used to create stillness while practicing the asanas. It helps to counteract distractions, anxious feelings, social awkwardness and negative energy.

Meditation during each restoratice yoga pose engages the mind-body unification practice that defines yoga as a whole.

Alignment and Balance – Props

Props are very important in restorative yoga. Yoga props assist physically in reaching your yoga goals. By utilizing props in your yoga practice, you are less likely to say, "I can't!"

We've all said or heard the "I can't do it" comments when it comes to yoga.

"I'm just not that flexible."

"I can't do yoga because I'm overweight."

"I'm too old."

"I had surgery years ago and just can't move the way I used to."

The best response to anyone justifying there inability to practice yoga is, "YES! You can."

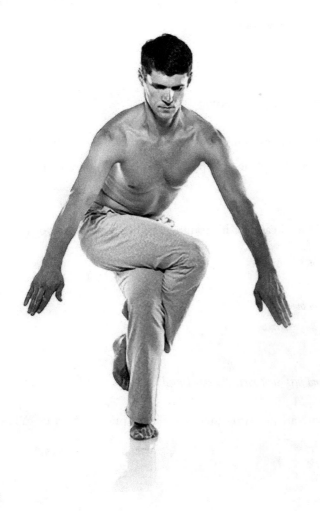

Yoga isn't about practicing like everyone else. Yoga isn't about looking like the girl or guy online or in the health and fitness books.

Yoga is simply practicing like YOU practice.

There is no one human body made exactly like the other. Your hand may not reach the floor during the Side Angle pose. That's ok! You may need a yoga block under your neck during Savasana to ease your lower back pain. Maybe rolling a blanket and placing it under you knees for spine support is necessary. There is no right or wrong way to practice yoga. It's all ok!

Everyone is different.

You are unique and so shall your yoga practice be!

Restorative yoga incorporates many different props that hav different responsibilities. They are there to aide your body's alignment and balance as your move through each pose.

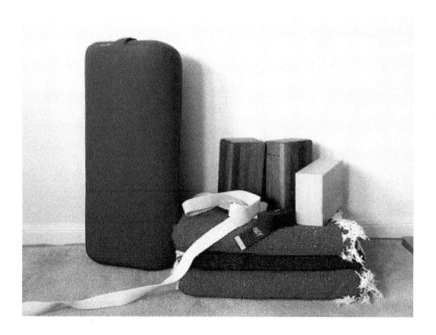

One important thing to remember when adding a prop to your pose, be patient. We may feel like we need to rush to grab a prop before trying a new pose. It's not important how quickly you get into the pose. Take your time. Listen first as the teacher explains the elements of the pose. Then decide whether or not you will need a prop based on how your body reacts to each movement.

If you need to come out of the pose to grab a prop, then do so. If your neck is straining, don't throw your shoulder out trying to reach the block or the blanket.

Be patient with your body. Utilizing a prop should create physical and mental relaxation, not added stress.

So, what in the world are these "props" we keep mentioning. Ok, let's see what all of these crazy blocks, straps and bolsters are all about!

Blocks

Yoga blocks are made of wood, foam or cork. These blocks can support your body in many of the yoga poses. For example, you can place the block next to you during a Side Angle or Triangle pose. This allows your to place your hand on the block instead of the floor. A block can also be used as a head rest during Savasana or under your lower back during Bridge pose.

Bolster

The bolster prop is most widely used in restorative yoga. This is a reactangular cushion providing support for many heart-opening and lower back exercises. The bolster can be used under the forehead during Child's pose or under the knees in Tree Top pose.

Straps

Straps are like large rubber bands used in many "stretch" poses. They act as extensions of the arm or leg for poses such as the Dancer pose or the Wheel pose. Straps can be used during a forward fold by wrapping it around your wrists and feet assisting in the stretch.

Sandbags

Sandbags are like large bean bags used to add weight on the body for a deeper stretch. They can be used on the hips during poses such as the Supine Twist

Blanket

Blankets in yoga have many different uses. You can use a blanket as your practice mat, folded as a cushion for an elbow or a knee, or as a pillow for your head during restorative poses.

Eye Pillow

The yoga eye pillow is used to block out light and helps to calm the brain. It facilitates a deeper meditation and filter out visual distractions. It is perfect for Savasana and can sometime be scented for aromatherapy.

Mat

The yoga mat is where it all happens. Your mat can be most anything that feels comfortable to you. Some use the typical foam mat that rolls up and is easy to carry. Some yoga students like to use blankets, or a"serape." Just make sure that whatever you choose offers support, stability and comfort.

Essential Oils

Aromatherapy changes the game! There's certainly nothing wrong with a little sweat during your yoga practice. But, when it's time to relax and soothe, choosing the right essential oil scent is important. Scents such as lavender, jasmine, sage, lemongrass and vanilla are all very popular in the restorative yoga practice.

Music

Set the tone with relaxing tunes. In a world of digital downloads, it's simple and easy to add music as you flow through each restorative yoga pose.

Yoga Flow

Flow yoga is a term that relates to a style of yoga focusing on patterned breathing and rhythmic movement.

Flowing through yoga is a beautiful movement. There are thousands of poses and many different sequences. That's why choosing your favorite type of yoga is a good decision. You can focus on practicing and developing the seqences or "flow" that works best for you and your body.

Yoga flow teach the body and the mind to work harmoniously together. Not only are you placing your body into specific poses, but your mind is learning to transition through to the next pose. This requires a reorganization of the mind, giving the brain a mental boost. Practicing continuous physical movement changes our thought patterns.. It helps us to get out of a rut sometimes. It also helps to boost our energy by bring on new challenges. When we train our brain to reorganize, we create a wealth of new thoughts and ideas.

Increasing mental focus and training our bodies to become stronger and more agile is very important at any age in life. Yoga flow is a low impact method used to gain strength of the mind and the body. The series of poses in a "flow" exercise, utilizes rhythmic breathing. It's very important to calculate each movement and whether or not you should be inhaling or exhaling at the same time. Your breath pattern is used to measure how long you will hold the pose. It also helps us to count through each movements during the same pose.

The process of patterned breathing while moving through a yoga sequence has many physical benefits. Breathing patterns can stabilize your heart rate, regulate body temperature and help you to maintain consistent movement all the way to the end of the exercise. Synchronizing your breath stables your heart rate and assists your body in releasing a balanced amount of heat. Therefore, your muscles will stretch and loosen properly during each exercise.

Learning yoga flow can be easy. The most important first step is to sign up for a class taught by a certified or qualified yoga instructor. It may be a good idea to initially choose a smaller class, especially if you are a true beginner in the yoga world. This way the instructor will have the time to address each student on a more personal level. He or she will have the chance to monitor your movemements. They can also personally assist you in modifying the pose based on your ability.

Attending a smaller class will also give you the opportunity to assess the space. Where should you place your mat? How much space will you need? Where are the props? Yoga flow classes also require intense focus. A smaller class can lessen the stress of unwanted distractions such as cramped space, the lack of props, phone noises, foot traffic, etc.

Obviously, the poses that you can expect in your Yoga Flow class depend on the level of the class.

Yoga levels are pretty basic – Beginner, Intermediate and Advanced. The instructor will most likely progress through a series of the same poses over a certain period of clases. Make sure to inquire about which level that you will be signing up for. There may be certain poses, positions, bends, stretches, etc. that could cause injury if you are not ready. This is true especially for back bends and inversion poses.

Yoga is a process. Everything you learn in your beginner class sets the foundation for your practice in the intermediate and advanced classes. So, sign up for that beginner class and plan to perfect the easy poses.

Your body will thank you.

The Many Types of Yoga

Hatha

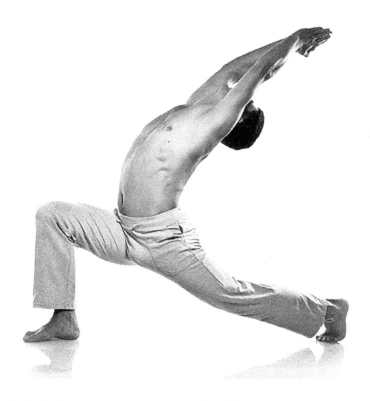

Hatha is the yoga practice that specifically deals with physical poses. Hatha is very common in Western culture. When people think of yoga, the physical poses immediately come to mind.

Hatha poses are slower and the movements are very calming. Yoga flow is integrated into a Hatha practice.

Also though the poses are slower and more relaxed, your body and mind still benefit from the poses. By flowing through the poses at a more relaxed pace, you can also focus on your breathing techniques and alignment during each movement. Hatha is a great practice for beginners.

Iyengar

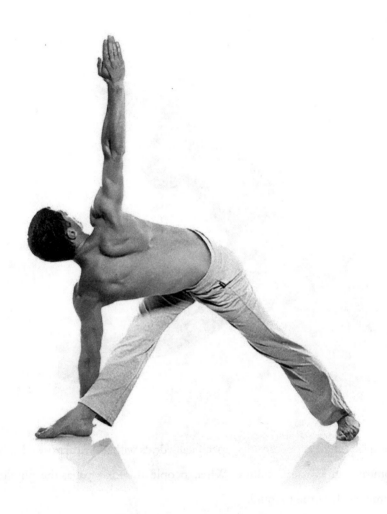

Iyengar was the man's name who founded Iyengar yoga. He was a very influential teacher in the yoga community.

Proper alignment and balance are the focus in Iyengar yoga. Poses are held for longer periods of time. Props such as mats, blocks and straps etc. are typically used in this practice. Poses are also be held longer in Hatha. Holding the poses for a longer period of time allow for a deeper stretch in order to promote the elongation of the muscles.

Iyengar promotes wellness of the mind and strong focus when moving into each pose. If you are dealing with an injury, this yoga practice allows you to pinpoint that specific area of your body to promote healing. And Iyengar instructor teaches the many aspects of each pose. He or she may note how each movement benefits a specific muscle.

You probably won't break a sweat during an Iyengar class either. Instead, each practice should end with mental clarity and relaxed muscles.

Bikram

You will definitely sweat in a Bikram yoga style class!

Bikram yoga was named after Bikram Choudhury. He developed this yoga style by turning the heat up in the room during class. Sometimes people refer to Bikram as "hot yoga." However, they are two different types of yoga.

Bikram yoga practices the same 26 poses in every class. You will practice those poses over and over again, learning and perfecting each one. The purpose of Bikram yoga is to loosen the muscles by working in a heated atmosphere.

If you plan to attend a Bikram yoga class, consult your instructor if you have been diagnosed with any ailment or sickness. You may need to modify the routine or take short breaks if you begin to feel short of breath or neasous. The temperature in a Bikram class can reach up to 104 degrees. Drink a lot of water, bring a towel and wear clothes that can withstand a heavy amount of sweat.

Ashtanga

K. Pattabhi Jois. brought Ashtanga yoga into the Western culture in the 1970's.

Ashtanga yoga focuses on consistent breathing and movement. This practice teaches you to connect a breathing pattern to the sequence of poses as directed by the instructor. It's purpose is continuous movement while following a very strenuous pace during the poses.

The yoga sequence is the same in each class. It's recommended to sign up for a few beginner classes before committing to an Ashtanga class. This way, you will become more familiar with the simple poses so that you can implement the more difficult poses during each sequence. Ashtanga yoga is designed to keep you moving.

Vinyasa

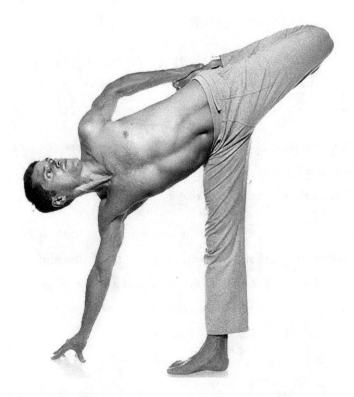

Vinyasa means to "place something in a special way."

Vinyasa is very similar to Restorative and Ashtanga yoga. The poses are held for a longer period of time. You are given more time to spend placing your body into the correct posture. With each breath, you are able to correct your alignment and balance.

Vinyasa incorporates yoga flow. While each pose is held for a longer period of time, you will still move continuously into the next pose. Depending on the instructor, the poses will most likely change with each class.

Focus is very important in a Vinyasa class. You will need to watch the instructor intently to make sure you are moving correctly into the next position. Although the pace may be slow, it is certainly continuous and can be energized with music.

Yin

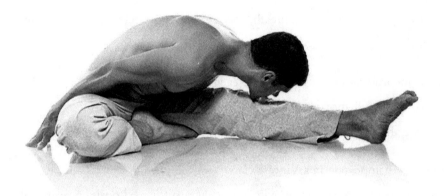

Yin is a great class for beginners. In a Yin class, you are given ample amount of time to perfect the poses for proper alignment and balance. You are also in a seated position to hold the poses for 2-5 minutes or more. It's not uncommon in a Yin class to complete only 3-5 poses within an hour. By holding the poses, Yin provides a "stretch to the bone."

This type of stretch not only stretches the muscles, but also loosens and releases the deep connective tissues. These stretch methods provide deeply relaxed muscles by the end of the class.

Meditation is also heavily integrated into a Yin practice. Since it is a slow-paced and quiet atmosphere, the student can integrate meditation into each pose.

Props are utilized in a Yin class as well. Props such as straps and blocks act as extensions of the limbs and provide a deeper stretch. This improves flexibility over time.

Restorative

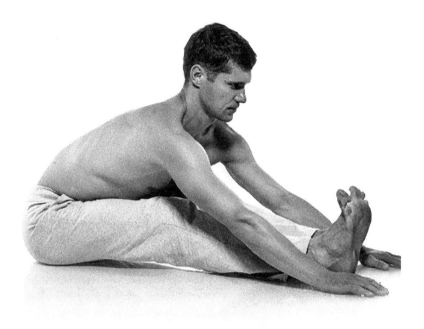

Ah, Restorative yoga. This level of a yoga practice is typically forgotten, especially in Western culture. We live in a "go-go-go" world and rarely get the option or the ability to slow down.

Most yoga classes will twist and turn your body into those pretzel poses as seen in the books and online. Not Restorative yoga. Restorative-style yoga relaxes and loosens your muscles. This practive gives you the chance to slow down and enter into a peaceful and calm mode of true rest.

Restorative yoga is best practiced in a dark, noiseless and open space. Find space that invites positive feelings and relaxing vibes. Whether your are signing up for a class at the gym or practicing at home, choose the best time of day that works for you. Obviously, make sure that you feel safe in the environment and void of any distractions. Your restorative space should be free of loud noises, cell phones tings and pings and negative energy.

Each pose in restorative yoga session should be used to relax your body. Everyone's body is different. Therefore, your restorative yoga practice should be designed to best fit the way that your body moves and stretches.

Restorative yoga poses are based heavily on props for support. These props assist each part of the body as needed. Extra blankets can cushion areas with added pressure. Bolsters aide in aligning the body and relieving painful stretchs. Straps act as extensions of the arms and legs allowing you to fasten the pose. Blocks support the neck, the back and the knees. Block can also act as landing pieces for hands and feet. You can add as many blankets as needed, folded or unfolded, to support any part of the body.

The great thing about restorative yoga is that you have time! Time to move into the position that feels best for you and your body. You have time to position a prop under, around or on top of your body for comfort.

Restorative is all about support. If your hand is dangling, or if your back is straining, grab a prop. Create your own support with the blocks, bolsters, blankets, etc. If your muscles are strained, they probably aren't being given proper support to ease into the restorative position.

Many times, this type of yoga calls for a very warm atmosphere. Some instructors will even lead you to grab an extra blanket for full body cover. Adding a weighted blanket to your body not only assists gravity in executing the pose, it also generates warmth for you're your muscles. The warmer your muscles are, the safer the stretch becomes.

Socks are also a good idea when practicing restorative yoga. In other yoga classes, you are usually instructed to practice with bare feet. However, in restorative yoga, as mentioned above, warmth is essential. Covering your feet in some form or fashion stops the release of body heat through the toes.

And, here's the kicker. You may fall asleep in a restorative yoga class. The goal is to not fall asleep. But, let's face it – warm air, relaxed muscles, blankets and a quiet room just might do the trick. It's ok. Your instructor will help to wake you properly and safely.

PART II

YOGA POSES

Beginner Poses

Hands to Heart

Sukhasana

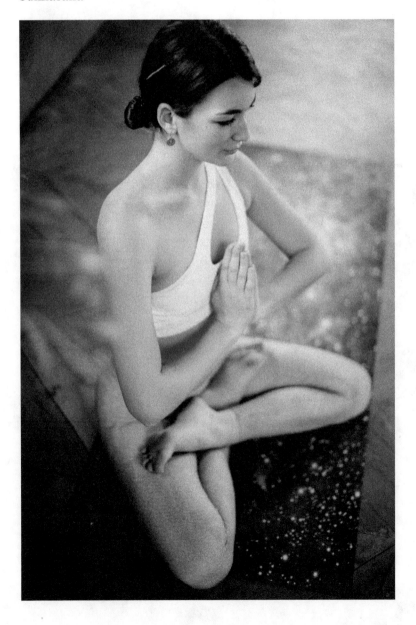

Level: Beginner

Position: Sitting

Style: Restorative, Stretch

Chakra: Root

Element: Earth Element

Anatomy Focus: Chest

In a seated position, cross your shins, widen your knees and slowly pull each foot onto the opposite thigh. Allow your knees to slowly relax towards the floor. Try not to force the movement. Let gravity do the work. Straighten your back and take a deep breath. Slowly exhale through your mouth. Place your hands together, palms touching, in front of your chest. Relax your shoulders and take another deep breath in and out through your mouth. Sukhasana can be practiced at the beginning as well as at the end of your yoga routine.

Tree

Vrksasana

Level: Beginner

Position: Standing

Style: Balance, Stretch, Strength

Chakra: Third Eye

Element: Light, Water, Earth

Anatomy Focus: Hamstrings, Hips, Knees, Quadriceps

Begin in a standing position, feet hip-width apart. Inhale and slowly bend one leg and place the bottom of the foot on the opposite inner thigh. Place your hands in Namaste, palms together in front of your chest. Exhale as you raise your hands above your head. Inhale and exhale. Gently bring your hands down to your side and lower your foot flat on the ground.

Standing   Variation

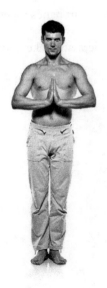
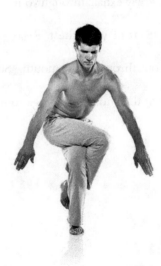

Staff

Dandasana

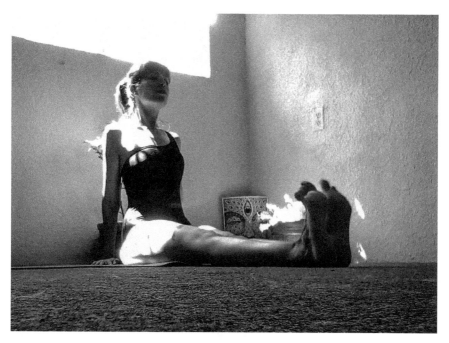

Level: Beginner

Position: Sitting

Style: Restorative, Stretch

Chakra: Solar Plexus, Sacral, Root

Element: Fire, Water, Earth

Anatomy Focus: Lower Back, Hips, Pelvis

In a seated position, inhale and exhale, straighten both legs in front of your body. Point both toes toward the sky and lower the back of both knees toward the floor. Straighten your spine, lower your shoulders and let the palms of your hands relax beside your hips. Practice breathing at a normal pace, loosening the leg muscles as you inhale and exhale.

Side Angle

Utthita Parsvakonasana

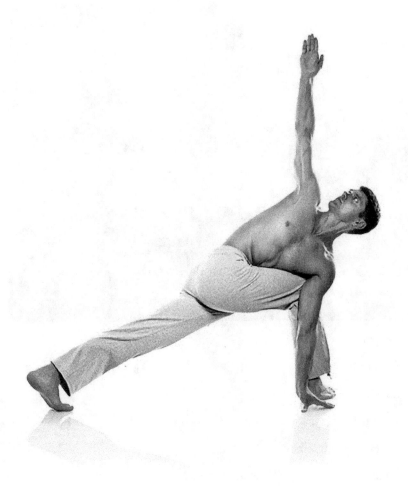

Level: Beginner

Position: Standing

Style: Side-Bend, Balance

Chakra: Heart, Sacral, Root

Element: Air, Water, Earth

Anatomy Focus: Arms and shoulders, Lower Back, Upper Back, Hamstrings, Chest, Hips, Knees, Pelvic, Psoas, Quadriceps

Begin this position in Star Pose. While rooted in Star Pose, point your right foot away from your body. Point your left foot forward, tighten your hips, engage your core and begin to bend your right knee. Inhale and exhale. Slowly shift your body to the right. As you bend, make sure that your knee is directly over your right foot. Adjust your left foot as needed to maintain balance and proper alignment. Bend your body to the right over your right knee and place your right hand firmly on the floor in front of your foot. Lift your left hand above your head and bring your gaze past your fingertips. Continue breathing normally and move back into Star pose. Keep both feet rooted firmly in the ground.

Downward Dog

Adho Mukha Svanasana

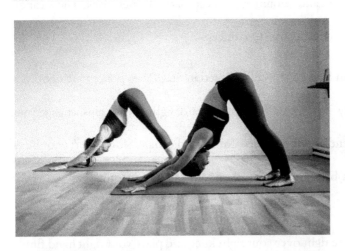

Level: Beginner

Position: Standing

Style: Inversion, Forward-Bend, Stretch, Strength

Chakra: Third Eye, Throat, Heart, Solar Plexus

Element: Light, Ether, Air, Fire

Anatomy Focus: Arms and Shoulders, Lower, Middle and Upper Back, Biceps and Triceps, Core, Feet and Ankles, Hamstrings

Begin in a standing position and lower your hands to the ground, palms placed firmly on the mat. Walk your hands out to 45 degree angle. Inhale and exhale, engaging your core and lowering your neck and head toward the mat. Turn your gaze in between your legs as you place your chin to your chest. Tighten the stomach muscles as you continue to inhale and exhale at a steady pace. Continue pointing your lower body toward the sky as you relax into the position. Inhale and exhale walking your hands back toward your body and slowly roll up to a standing position.

Upward Facing Dog

Urdhva Mukha Svanasana

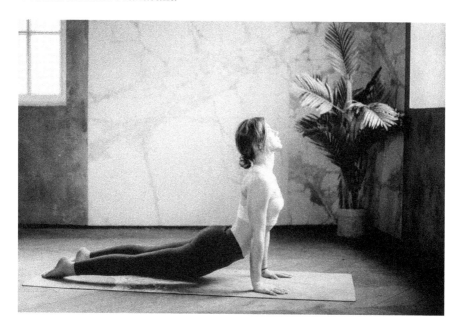

Level: Beginner

Position: Prone

Style: Back-bend, Stretch, Strength

Chakra: Throat, Heart, Solar Plexus, Sacral, Root

Element: Ether, Air, Fire, Water, Earth

Anatomy Focus: Arms and Shoulders, Lower and Middle Back, Biceps and Triceps, Core, Chest, Neck, Pelvic, Psoas

Start your pose in a prone position on your mat. Relax the stomach muscles. Inhale and exhale. Place both palms flat in front of you with your elbows bent. Press both thighs onto your mat and slowly press your hands down and lift your chest. Continue to inhale and exhale lifting until your arms and straighten your elbow. Keep both arms close to your body. Let your feet relax as you ease into the pose, breathing at a continuous pace. Slowly bend your elbows and lower your chest back down to your mat.

Thunderbolt

Vajrasana

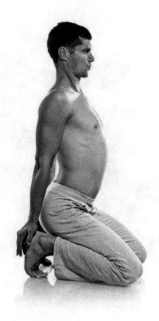

Level: Beginner

Position: Sitting

Style: Stretch

Chakra: Third Eye, Sacral, Root

Element: Light, Water, Earth

Anatomy Focus: Feet and Ankles, Knees

In a seated position, straighten both legs out in front of your body. Inhale and exhale, straightening your spine, lowering both shoulders and tightening your core muscles. Gently bend your left leg behind your body so that your foot meets your gluteus. Repeat the same movement with your right leg. Let your buttocks relax down onto both feet and place your palms on both quadriceps. Close your eyes and continue to breath at a steady pace relaxing your upper body with each inhale and exhale.

Child's

Balasana

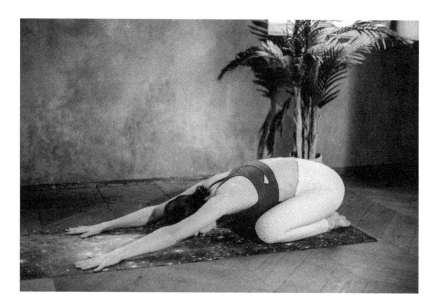

Level: Beginner

Position: Prone

Style: Restorative, Forward-Bend, Inversion

Chakra: Crown, Third Eye, Solar Plexus, Sacral, Root

Element: Thought, Light, Fire, Water, Earth

Anatomy Focus: Lower Back, Feet and Ankles, Hips, Knees, Neck

Begin by sitting in the Thunderbolt Pose. Raise your buttocks, widen your feet and lower your buttocks back down to the floor. Keep your calves and feet close to the body. Inhale and exhale folding forward and placing your forehead gently on your mat. Continue to inhale and exhale moving your arms behind you resting them next to your thighs. Palms facing up, allow both shoulders to slowly drift toward the mat. Continue breathing at a normal pace in this position and then slowly return to a seated Thunderbolt pose.

Warrior I

Virabhadrasana I

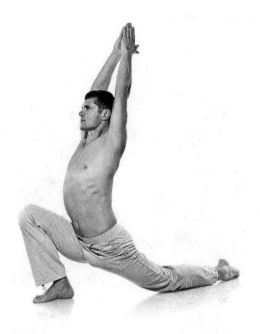

Level: Beginner

Position: Standing

Style: Stretch, Twist, Strength

Chakra: Throat, Heart, Solar Plexus, Sacral, Root

Element: Ether, Air, Fire, Water, Earth

Anatomy Focus: Lower and Middle Back, Hamstrings, Chest, Hips, Knees, Neck, Psoas, Quadriceps

Begin in Mountain Pose. Inhale and exhale and step your right foot behind your body. Place it firmly on your mat at a 20 degree angle to create the proper balance. Bend your left leg in front of your body. Make sure that your knee is placed directly above the top of your foot. Lift both arms directly above your head placing your biceps close to your ears. Continue breathing at a normal pace. Lower both shoulders and shift your gaze past your fingertips. Slowly, bring your right leg back to meet your left leg, straighten your spine and lower both arms.

Warrior II

Virabhadrasana II

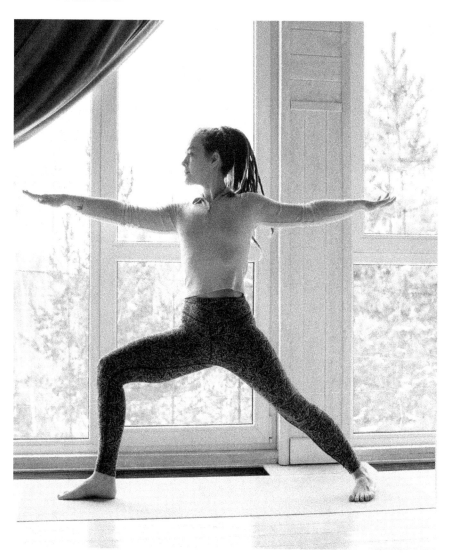

Level: Beginner

Position: Standing

Style: Stretch, Strength, Balance

Chakra: Sacral, Root

Element: Water, Earth

Anatomy Focus: Arms and Shoulders, Lower and Middle Back, Hamstrings, Chest, Hips, Knees, Psoas, Quadriceps

Begin in Mountain Pose. Inhale and exhale repositioning into Star Pose. Place both feet further than hip width apart and raise both arms to shoulder level. Point your palms down to the ground. Point your right foot away from the body and position your left foot facing forward. With your arms out wide, inhale and exhale tightening your core stomach muscles. Slowly shift your torso to the right, bending the right knee and placing it directly over the top of the foot. With a fluid movement, twist your upper body to the right and shift your gaze past your fingertips. Inhale and exhale reversing the movement to return to Star position. Gently move both feet to meet each other landing back in Mountain Pose.

Mountain

Tadasana

Level: Beginner

Position: Standing

Style: Restorative, Balance

Chakra: Sacral, Root

Element: Water, Earth

Anatomy Focus: Feet and Ankles

Standing with your feet together, straighten your spine and drop your hands to your hips. Let your shoulders relax, inhale and exhale. Engage your lower body, hips and core, pulling your navel softly toward your spine. Let your arms relax on either side of your body. Inhale through your nose and out through your mouth.

Star

Utthita Tadasana

Level: Beginner

Position: Standing

Style: Stretch

Chakra: Sacral, Root

Elements: Water, Earth

Anatomy Focus: Arms and Shoulders, Chest, Hips

Begin in Mountain Pose. Inhale and exhale widening your feet beyond hip distance. Position the soles of the feet flat on the floor. Make sure each toe is firmly placed on the ground. Lift your spine, lower both shoulders and engage your core. Tighten both legs and center the hips aligning the body for proper balance. Inhale and exhale at a normal pace and lift both arms to shoulder height. Point your fingers, palms facing downwards and lower your shoulders away from your ears. Continue breathing. Close your eyes if desired. Inhale and exhale letting your mind focus on the outward positioning while tightening your core at the same time.

Corpse

Savasana

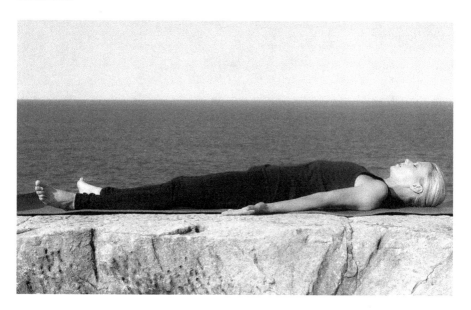

Level: Beginner

Position: Supine

Style: Restorative

Chakra: Crown, Heart

Elements: Thought, Air

Anatomy Focus: Lower Back

Begin in a seated position with both legs straight in front of your body. Lower both shoulders, tuck your lower back and place your chin to your chest. Reach both arms in front of your upper body. Inhale, exhale and slowly roll down to a supine position. Rest both arms wide beside your body with palms facing the sky. Let your feet fall the side. Allow the backs of your legs to loosen. Let your spine, neck and head melt into the mat as your breathing slows to a natural rhythm.

Butterfly

Baddha Konasana

Level: Beginner

Position: Sitting

Style: Stretch

Chakra: Sacral, Root

Element: Water, Earth

Anatomy Focus: Lower Back, Feet and Ankles, Hamstrings, Hips, Knees, Pelvic

In a seated position, lift your spine and straighent both legs in front of your body. Inhale and exhale. Bend both legs until the bottom of your feet are facing one another in front of your torso on your mat. Allow your legs to slowly relax into the seated position. Grip the each big toe with your hands. Inhale and exhale as you gently bend forward. Gaze down toward your toes. Continue inhaling and exhaling as you slowly straighten your spine back to your seated position.

Hero

Virasana

Level: Beginner

Position: Sitting

Style: Stretch

Chakra: Sacral, Root

Element: Water, Earth

Anatomy Focus: Hips, Knees, Quadriceps

Begin in Table Top position. Sit back on your buttocks resting in between both knees. Place both hands on your quadriceps, palms down. Inhale and gently lower your chin to your chest. Exhale and let your hips relax into the seated position. Continue to inhale and exhale making sure to keep your shoulders lowered and away from your ears.

Garland

Malasana

Level: Beginner

Position: Standing

Style: Stretch

Chakra: Sacral, Root

Element: Water, Earth

Anatomy Focus: Lower Back, Hamstrings, Hips, Pelvic

Begin in Mountain pose, lift your spine and engage your core. Bring your hands to Namaste, inhale and gently bend both knees lowering your buttocks to the floor. Balance on your feet and rest both elbows on your inner thighs. Inhale and exhale as you slowly place both palms on the floor to push back up to standing position. Continue breathing at a normal pace.

Cobbler

Baddha Konasana

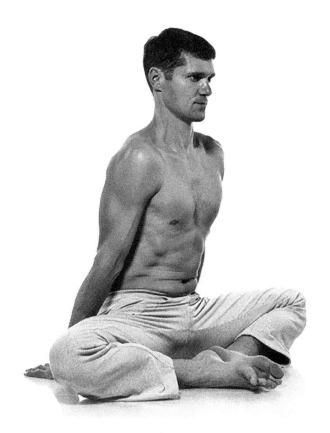

Level: Beginner

Position: Sitting

Style: Stretch

Chakra: Sacral, Root

Anatomy Focus: Lower Back, Feet and Ankles, Hamstrings, Hips, Knees, Pelvic

In a seated position, begin with your feet and legs in front of you. Inhale and exhale as you bend both knees until the bottom of your feet are touching. Allow both feet to relax on the floor and grasp each big toe firmly with your hands.

Inhale and exhale stretching both knees further toward the floor. Place both of your elbows on your thighs, bend forward gazing toward your feet. Inhale and exhale and lift your spine back to a seated position.

Chair

Utkatasana

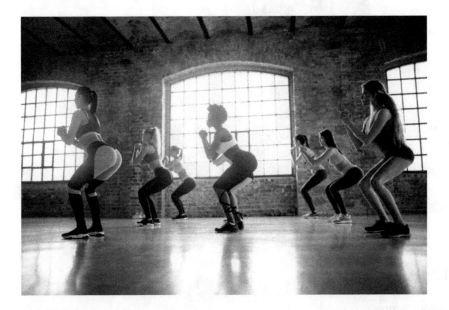

Level: Beginner

Position: Standing

Style: Forward-Bend, Stretch, Strength, Balance

Chakra: Throat, Sacral, Root

Element: Ether, Water, Earth

Anatomy Focus: Arms and Shoulders, Lower Back, Hips, Knees, Pelvic,

Quadriceps

Begin in Mountain pose. Move your feet together so that they are touching. Plant both feet firmly in the ground, focusing on the heels as well as each toe. Inhale and exhale engaging your core, lowering your shoulder and tightening the glute muscles. Bend both knees. Make sure the knees are positioned directly above the feet. Continue to inhale and exhale, lowering the buttocks slightly. Lift both arms above your head and let both biceps rest near your ears. Lower both shoulders and shift your gaze upward past your fingertips. Hold this position as you inhale and exhale. Allow the upper body to gently rest upon the lower body.

Cat

Marjaryasana

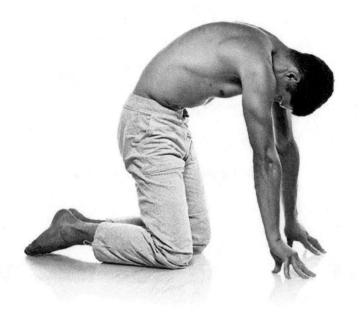

Level: Beginner

Position: Prone

Style: Forward-Bend

Chakra: Solar Plexus

Element: Fire

Anatomy Focus: Lower and Middle Back, Neck

In a seated position, move into Table Top Pose resting your body on your hands and knees. Inhale and exhale and tighten your stomach muscles. Position your feet behind you and place both palms firmly on the mat. Engage each fingertip for the proper balance and alignment. Inhale and curve your back upwards, pulling your stomach in toward the spine. Tuck your chin to your chest, relax your shoulders and exhale. Lower your back to its resting Table Top position. Continue this movement inhaling and exhaling rounding your back and loosening the back muscles.

Cow

Bitilasana

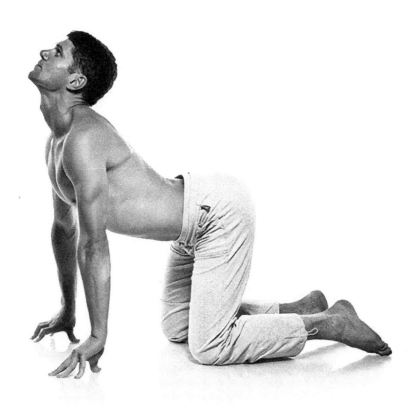

Level: Beginner

Position: Prone

Style: Back-Bend

Chakra:

Element:

Anatomy Focus: Lower Back, Knees, Neck

In a seated position, move into Table Top Pose resting your body on your hands and knees. Inhale and exhale while tightening your stomach muscles. Position your feet behind you and place both palms firmly on the mat. Engage each fingertip for the proper balance and alignment. Inhale and bring your stomach toward the floor and curving the back into a U-shape. Lift your chin and stretch your neck and face toward the sky. Lower both shoulders and exhale. Return to table Top position. Continue this movement with slow deep breaths to release tension in the lower back muscles.

Side Lunge

Skandasana

Level: Beginner

Position: Sitting

Style: Stretch, Balance

Chakra: Sacral, Root

Element: Water, Earth

Anatomy Focus: Feet and Ankles, Hamstrings, Hips, Knees, Pelvic, Quadriceps

The Side Lunge can begin in Mountain Pose or continued from the Low Lunge pose. Slowly lower your body to the floor, supporting yourself with both hands and fingertips in front you on your mat. As you lower down, bend your right leg and rest your inner thigh on the top of your right heel. Point your left leg straight out to the side of your body resting your heel on the floor, left toes pointing to the sky. Continue inhaling and exhaling engaging your stomach muscles, lowering your shoulders and tightening your glutes.

Sphinx

Niravalasana

Variation

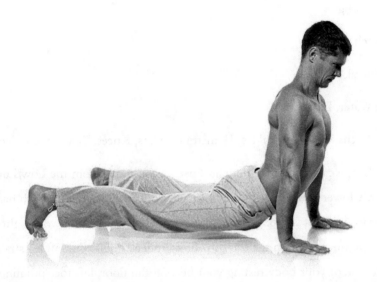

Level: Beginner

Position: Prone

Style: Back-Bend

Chakra:

Element:

Anatomy Focus: Lower Back, Biceps and Triceps, Chest

Begin in prone position. Bend both elbows keeping them close to your body, palms pushing into your mat. Keep both feet together and gently push your upper body off of your mat utilizing the triceps. Make sure to relax your neck, inhaling and exhaling during the entire stretch. Feel your stomach muscles engage toward your mat with each breath. Slowly lower back down to your met.

High Lunge

Ashta Chandrasana

Level: Beginner

Position: Standing

Style: Stretch, Strength, Balance

Chakra: Sacral, Root

Element: Water, Earth

Anatomy Focus: Arms and Shoulders, Lower and Upper Back, Hamstrings, Hips, Knees, Psoas, Quadriceps

From Downward Dog or Mountain Pose, lift both arms above your head keeping them close to your ears. Relax the shoulders. Bend your left knee and step your right foot behind your body landing on your toes. Make sure your left knee is directly above the top of the foot. And, keep your right knee slightly bent with the weight on the bottom of your right foot. Inhale and exhale continuously. Tuck your torso and engage your core on the exhale. Step your right foot forward to meet your left foot, returning to Mountain pose.

Supine Twist

Supta Matsyendrasana

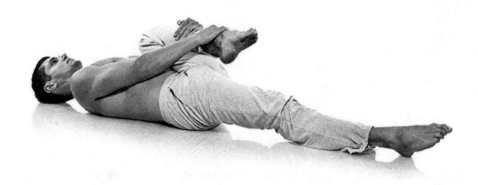

Level: Beginner

Position: Supine

Style: Twist, Stretch

Chakra: Sacral, Root

Element: Water, Earth

Anatomy Focus: Lower and Middle Back, Hamstrings, Hips, Knees, Neck

Begin by laying down flat on your back. Inhale and bend both knees into your chest. Flatten your lower back into the floor and relax both shoulders. Gently begin to drop both knees to one side of your body, relaxing one knee on top of the other. Lay both arms out wide and shift your gaze in the opposite direction. Inhale and exhale continuously through this stretch. Slowly bring both knees back to your chest and lower down to your mat.

Legs up the Wall

Viparita Karani

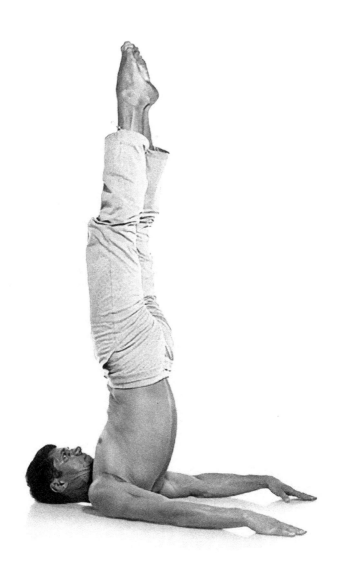

Level: Beginner

Position: Supine

Style: Restorative, Stretch

Chakra:

Element:

Anatomy Focus: Lower Back, Pelvic, Quadriceps

Find an empty wall away from mirrors or windows. Begin in supine position with both knees bent. Move your buttocks against the wall with both hands down by your side. Inhale and exhale, placing both legs flat against the wall. Relax your neck and lower back into the floor. Breath continuously through this pose allowing the blood to begin flowing in a different direction.

Sitting Forward Fold

Paschimottanasana

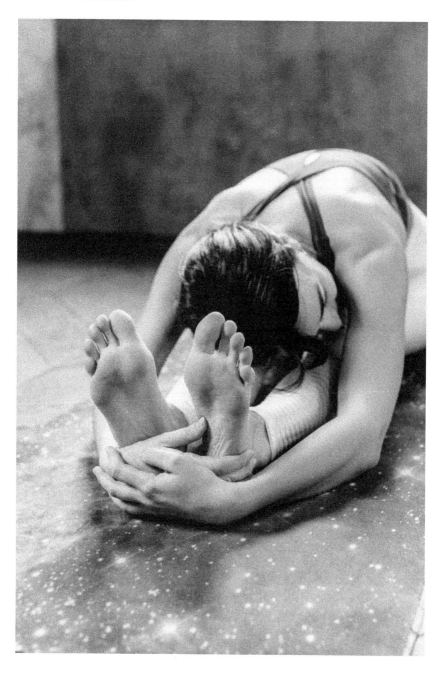

Level: Beginner

Position: Sitting

Style: Forward-Bend, Stretch

Chakra: Throat, Solar-Plexus, Root

Element: Ether, Fire, Water, Earth

Anatomy Focus: Lower and Upper Back, Hamstrings, Hips, Neck

While in Staff pose, inhale and tuck your chin to your chest. Engage your core and lower both shoulders. Beginning to create a curve at the top of your neck. Slowly roll forward one vertebrae at a time. Keeping both hands by your side for support, palms down. Roll down as far as your spine will allow without forcing the motion. Slowly roll back up returning to Staff pose.

Standing Forward Fold

Uttanasana

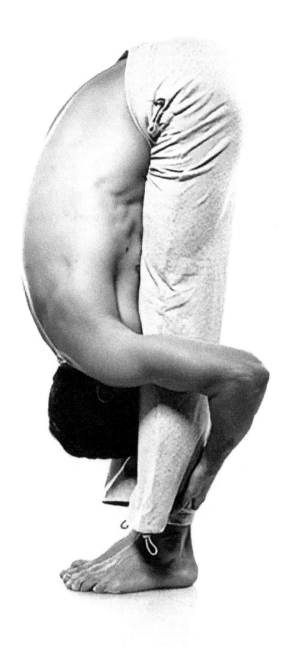

Level: Beginner

Position: Standing

Style: Forward-Bend, Stretch, Inversion

Chakra: Crown, Solar-Plexus, Sacral, Root

Element: Thought, Fire, Water, Earth

Anatomy Focus: Lower and Upper Back, Hamstrings, Hips, Neck

Begin in Mountain pose. Inhale, tuck your chin to your chest and lower both shoulders. Exhale and slowly roll down one vertebrae at a time gazing toward your toes. Allow gravity to assist with the stretch. Try not to force or push the stretch as you fold. Slowly roll back up, chin to chest, returning to Mountain pose.

Table Top

Bharmanasana

Level: Beginner

Position: Sitting

Style: Restorative

Chakra: Sacral, Root

Element: Water, Earth

Anatomy Focus: Arms and Shoulders, Lower Back, Biceps and Triceps, Knees

In Vajrasana, walk both hands out in front of your body stopping just below the shoulders. Lift up on your knees. Keep both feet on the floor. Inhale and exhale engaging your stomach muscles. Align your head and neck with your back so that your upper torso is parallel to your mat. Shift your gaze to the mat. Gently rotate back into Child's pose.

Plank

Phalakasana

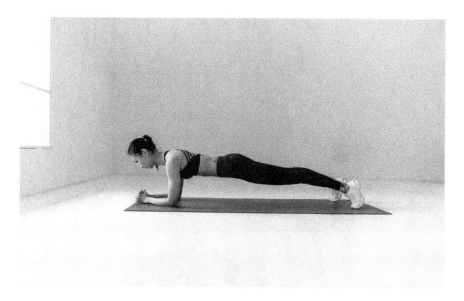

Level: Beginner

Position: Prone

Style: Strength

Chakra: Solar Plexus

Element: Fire

Anatomy Focus: Arms and Shoulders, Biceps and Triceps, Core

In Downward Dog pose, plant both feet and hands firmly on your mat, utilizing all fingertips for balance. Slowly move the entire body parallel to your mat focusing weight on the toes and hands. Make sure both hands are directly below both shoulders. Inhale and exhale through each move. Gaze toward the floor shifting the hips inward. If your wrists begin to experience a painful pressure, release to your elbows keeping your hands in front of your body. Inhale and exhale. Gently fold back to Child's pose when ready.

Bridge

Setubandha Sarvangasana

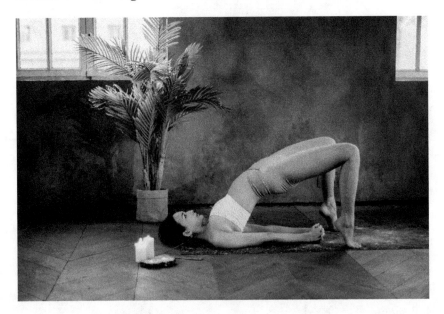

Level: Beginner

Position: Supine

Style: Back-Bend, Stretch, Strength, Balance

Chakra: Crown, Third Eye, Throat, Solar Plexus

Element: Thought, Light, Ether, Fire

Anatomy Focus: Arms and Shoulders, Lower and Upper Back, Core, Chest, Hips, Neck, Pelvic, Psoas, Quadriceps

Begin this pose in supine position. Bend both knees bringing them close to your buttocks. Place both hands by your side, palms down. Inhale and exhale, lifting the buttocks off the floor by pushing through the soles of the feet. Make sure to support your neck by keeping it flat on the mat. Lift through to your toes if desired. Slowly lower back down to your mat.

Camel

Ustrasana

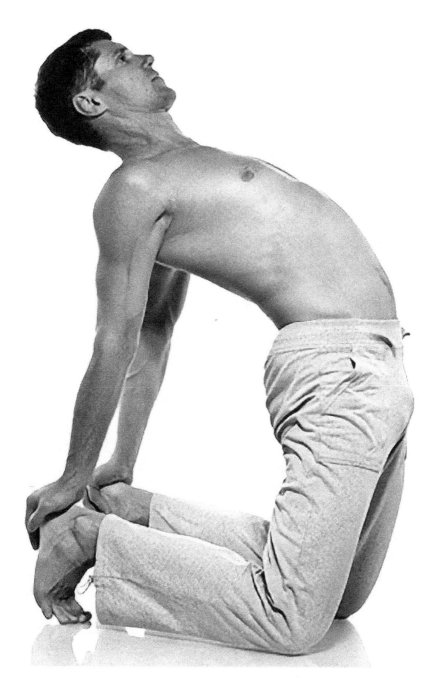

Level: Beginner

Position: Sitting

Style: Back-Bend, Stretch, Balance

Chakra: Crown, Third-Eye, Throat, Heart, Solar-Plexus

Element: Thought, Light, Ether, Air, Fire

Anatomy Focus: Lower, Middle and Upper Back, Core, Chest, Knees, Neck, Pelvic, Psoas, Quadriceps

While in Thunderbolt Pose, lift to your knees, straighten your spine and lower both shoulders. Slowly place both palms behind your body, on top of each respective heel. Open the chest, inhale, and rotate back, supporting the neck. Shift your gaze toward the sky, inhale and exhale. Tightening the quadriceps, rotate back to Thurnderbolt pose.

Four Limbed Staff Pose

Chaturanga Dandasana

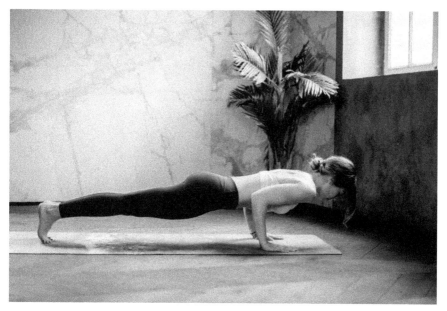

Level: Beginner

Position: Prone

Style: Strength

Chakra: Solar Plexus

Element: Fire

Anatomy Focus: Arms and Shoulders, Lowers Back, Biceps and Triceps, Core, Hamstrings, Pelvic

Begin this pose in Downward Dog and walk into Plank Pose. Find the correct balance on your toes and palms of your hands while gazing toward the floor. Take a few deep breaths, tighten your core muscles and slowly bend both elbows by your side, keeping them as close your body as possible. As you lower, keep your body parallel to the floor and exhale. Breathing continuously, push up through your palms, lower both knees and sit back into Child's Pose.

Cobra

Bhujangasana

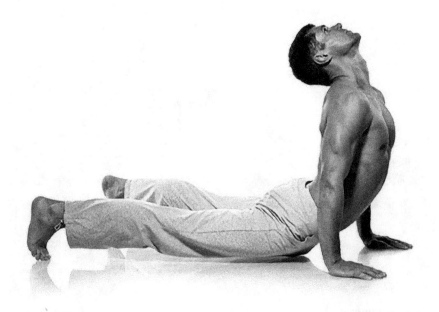

Level: Beginner

Position: Prone

Style: Back-Bend

Chakra: Throat, Heart, Solar Plexus, Sacral, Root

Element: Ether, Air, Fire, Water, Earth

Anatomy Focus: Lower, Middle and Upper Back, Biceps and Triceps, Core, Psoas

Lying on your stomach in prone position with face down, inhale and exhale tightening the stomach muscles. Firmly plant the top of your feet to the ground and place your palms close to your upper abdomen. Inhale and push through your palms, raising your chest about six inches off the ground. Exhale. Slowly lower down to your mat.

Intermediate Poses

Seated Twist

Marichyasana

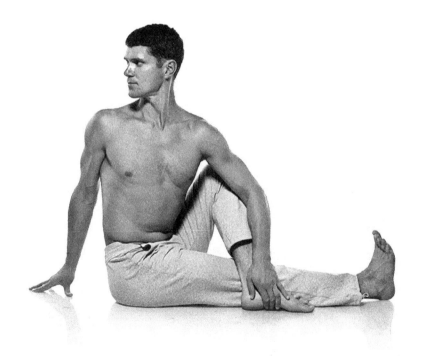

Level: Intermediate

Position: Sitting

Style: Twist, Forward-Bend, Stretch

Chakra: Solar, Sacral, Root

Element: Fire, Water, Earth

Anatomy Focus: Arms and Shoulders, Lower and Upper Back, Biceps and Triceps, Core, Hamstrings, Hips, Neck, Quadriceps

Begin in Staff Pose with feet straight out in front of your body. Inhale and exhale as your lift your right leg toward your chest. Keep your left leg straight, inhale and twist your torso as you place your left hand on the floor behind you. Bring your right arm around your right knee and slowly bend forward. Gently lift both hands behind you and lock them together. Inhale and exhale as you lower into the final position. Slowly release your hands and return to your upright seated position.

Boat

Navasana

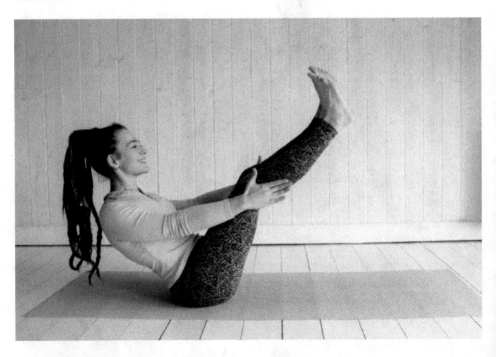

Level: Intermediate

Position: Sitting

Style: Forward Bend, Strength, Balance

Chakra: Solar Plexus

Element: Fire

Anatomy Focus: Lower Back, Core, Pelvic, Quadriceps

Begin in a seated position, inhale and exhale, pointing both legs out in front of your body. Slowly round your spine and engage your core muscles. Turn your gaze toward your knees. Inhale and exhale as you bring your legs 1-2 feet off the ground in a straight motion. Point your toes. Raise both arms and place your hands, palms facing in, to the outside of your knees. Inhale and exhale as your bring your arms and legs down slowly to the ground.

Wheel

Chakrasana

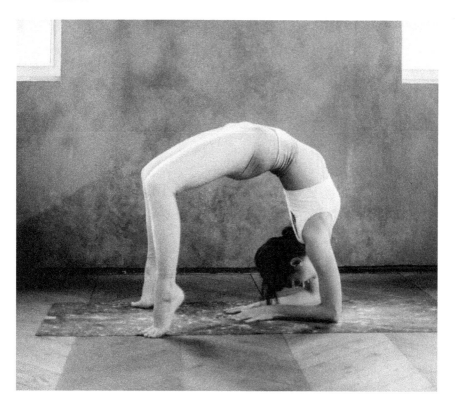

Level: Intermediate

Position: Supine

Style: Back-Bend, Stretch, Inversion, Strength, Balance

Chakra: Crown, Third Eye, Throat, Heart, Solar Plexus

Element: Thought, Light, Ether, Air, Fire

Anatomy Focus: Lower Back, Core, Chest, Neck, Psoas, Quadriceps

Begin in Corpse pose, a supine position. Bring the focus to your lower back and bend both knees placing the feet flat on the floor. Inhale and exhale and place both hands behind your head, palms on the floor. Point fingers toward the shoulders and rotate both wrists away from your body. Inhale. As you exhale, slowly lift your torso off the floor. Make sure to balance the weight of your body on both the palms of your hands as well as on the soles of both feet. Continue a normal breathing pattern as you find your comfort level. Set your gaze past your elbows in this position. Slowly lower your torso down the ground. Inhale and exhale returning to the supine position.

Warrior III

Virabhadrasana III

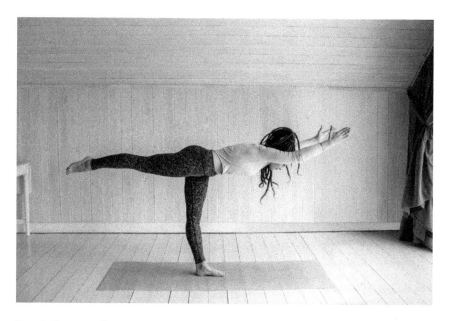

Level: Intermediate

Position: Standing

Style: Balance, Forward-Bend, Stretch, Strength, Balance

Chakra: Solar Plexus, Sacral, Root

Element: Fire, Water, Earth

Anatomy Focus: Middle Back, Core, Hamstrings, Chest, Hips, Psoas, Quadriceps

Begin in Mountain Pose. Inhale and exhale repositioning into Star Pose, feet further than hip width apart and arms raised to shoulder level. Point your palms down to the ground. Point your right foot away from the body and position your left foot facing forward. With your arms out wide, inhale and exhale tightening your core stomach muscles. Slowly shift your torso to the right, bending the right knee and placing it directly over the top of the foot. With a fluid movement, twist your upper body to the right and shift your gaze past your fingertips. Bring your left arm parallel to your right arm, palms facing one another. Twist your entire body to the right, folding your head in between your biceps and lift your left leg off the ground. Point your left foot. Inhale and exhale tightening the stomach muscles. Shift your weight as need on your left leg to find the correct balance and alignment. Point the crown of your head toward the tips of your fingers. Hold this position for a few deep breaths. Lower yyour left leg, return both arms to your side and rest back into Mountain pose.

Triangle

Trikonasana

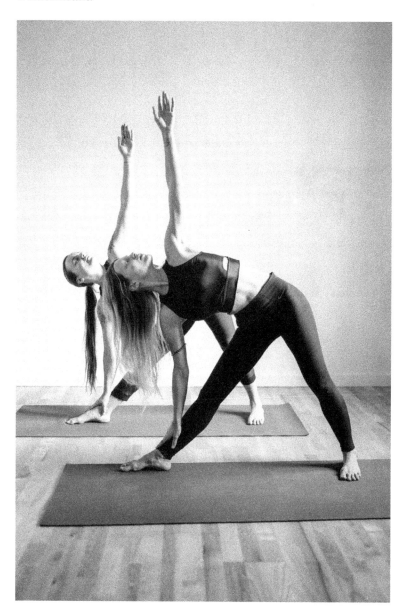

Level: Intermediate

Position: Standing

Style: Side-Bend, Stretch

Chakra: Heart, Sacral, Root

Element: Air, Water, Earth

Anatomy Focus: Arms and Shoulders, Biceps and Triceps, Core, Hamstrings, Chest, Psoas, Quadriceps

Begin in Star Pose, feet apart. Place both arms out wide, shoulder-width apart. Turn your right foot out 90 degrees and rotate your left foot forward. Inhale and exhale tightening your core and engaging your lower back muscles. Slightly rotate your lower back forward. With arms still placed out wide, slowly rotate down the right side of your body, fingers pointing toward your shin. Slowly lower your right hand to the floor behind your leg. Reach your left arm to the sky. Shift your gaze upward past your fingertips. Continue breathing through the pose. Slowly rotate back to Star Pose. Relax your arms to your sides and walk your feet together.

Plow

Halasana

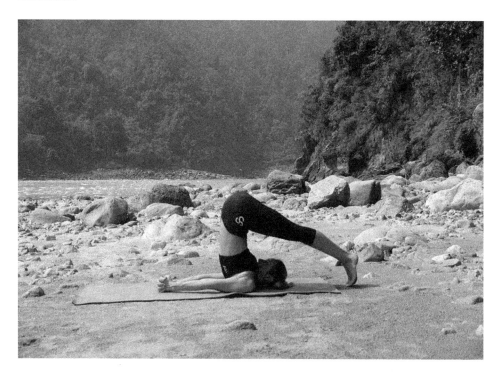

Level: Intermediate

Position: Supine

Style: Inversion, Stretch

Chakra: Crown, Third Eye, Throat, Solar Plexus

Element: Thought, Light, Ether, Fire

Anatomy Focus: Lower, Middle and Upper Back, Core, Hamstrings, Hips, Neck, Pelvic

Begin in supine position with both legs on the floor. Inhale and raise both legs to a 90 degree angle. Exhale pushing your arms and palms to the floor, rotate your legs completely over your head. Inhale and exhale as your toes touch the floor behind your head. Continue breathing through the pose. Lower both legs back to supine position.

Low Lunge

Parsva Anjaneyasana

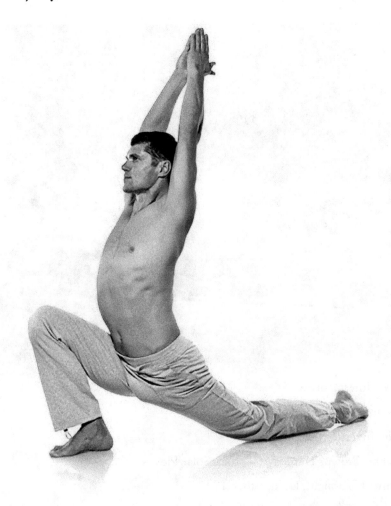

Level: Intermediate

Position: Sitting

Style: Side-Bend, Stretch, Strength, Balance

Chakra: Sacral, Root

Element: Water, Earth

Anatomy Focus: Arms and Shoulders, Upper Back, Biceps and Triceps, Core, Chest, Hips, Knees, Psoas, Quadriceps

Follow the steps from Warrior Pose II to move into a Low Lunge. Once in Warrior Pose II, raise both arms above your head and lower your right knee to the mat. Inhale and exhale resting the entire right leg straight behind your body. Let your knee rest gently on the mat. Your left knee should be directly above the top of your foot. Continue moving through the pose by lowering your shoulders and allowing your hips to drift slowly toward your mat stretching the hamstrings. If your knee begins to feel a painful pressure, place a blanket or mat underneath to add a cushion during this pose. Inhale and exhale. Move your right leg in front of your body, lower both arms and relax back into Child's Pose as needed.

Side Plank

Vasisthasana

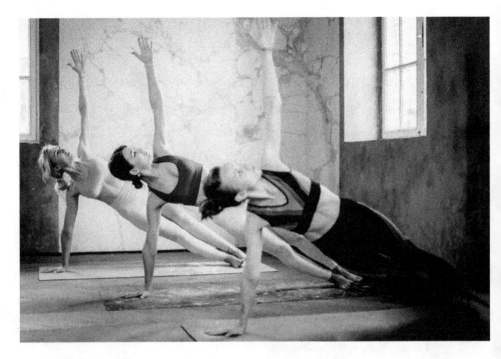

Level: Intermediate

Position: Sitting

Style: Balance, Stretch, Strength

Chakra: Solar Plexus

Element: Fire

Anatomy Focus: Arms and Shoulders, Biceps and Triceps, Core

Begin in Plank pose. Inhale and rotate your entire body to the right side. Lift your left arm to the sky and shift your gaze upward. Let your left foot rest firmly on your right foot. Push through your right palm for balance and alignment. Engage your stomach muscles to provide core support. Rotate back to Plank pose and sit back into Child's pose as needed.

Half Moon

Ardha Chandrasana

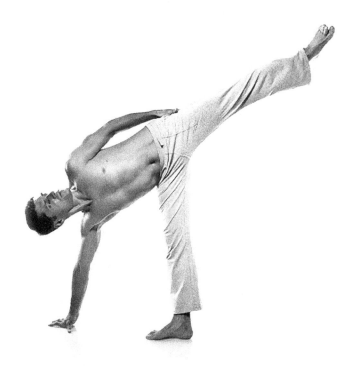

Level: Intermediate

Position: Standing

Style: Side-Bend, Inversion, Strength, Balance

Chakra: Sacral, Root

Element: Water, Earth

Anatomy Focus: Biceps and Triceps, Core, Hamstrings, Hips, Psoas, Quadriceps

Stand in Mountain Pose. Use a yoga block as needed. Place the block beside your mat within arm's reach. Spread both legs, turn your right foot to the right toward the block and point your left foot forward. Inhale and exhale and slowly lean to your right placing your right hand on the block, or on the floor. Raise your left leg so that it is parallel to your mat. Lift your left hand to the sky and shift your gaze past your fingertips. Return to Mountain Pose.

Dancer Pose

Natarajasana

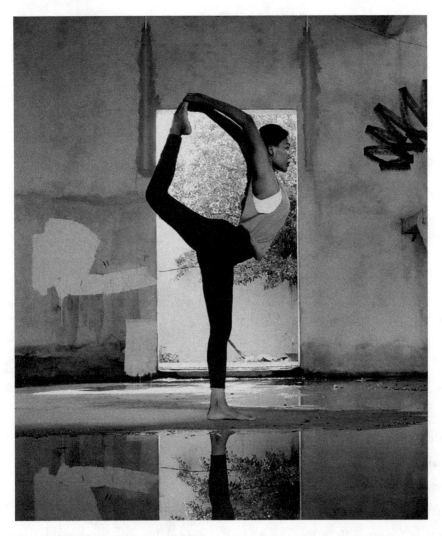

Level: Intermediate

Position: Standing

Style: Stretch, Back-Bend, Strength, Balance

Chakra: Heart, Solar-Plexus

Element: Air, Fir

Anatomy Focus: Lower Back, Biceps and Triceps, Hamstrings, Chest, Hips, Psoas, Quadriceps

Dancer Pose begins in Mountain Pose. Straighten your spine and bring your lower back slightly inward. Engage your core. Inhale and exhale bending the right knee letting the heel of your foot reach the buttocks. Stretch your right hand behind your body. Grab the toes of your right foot. Continue to inhale and exhale lifting your chest and tightening your stomach muscles. Reach your left hand straight out in front of your body. Take a deep breath in and out and twist your shoulders. Roll your fingers and thumb of your right hand around your big toe. Rotate the right elbow and shoulders allowing your arm to migrate above your head. Continue to stretch the left arm in front of you while maintaining your core balance. Plant your left foot firmly on your mat engaging the heel as well as each toe for proper balance and alignment. Slowly rotate your right arm over your head, releasing the right foot. Return to Mountain Pose.

Advanced Poses

Reclined Middle Split

Supta Trivikramasana

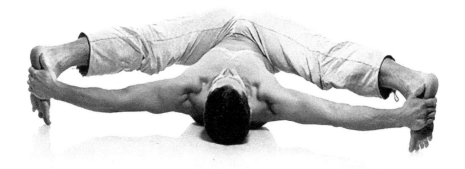

Level: Advanced

Position: Supine

Style: Stretch

Chakra: Sacral, Root

Element: Water, Earth

Anatomy Focus: Quadriceps

Begin seated in Staff Pose. Slowly roll onto your back. Inhale and exhale planting your left leg firmly on the mat. Raise your right leg to a 90 degree angle. Grasp the big right toe and rotate your right hip. Engage the stomach muscles on the exhale and bring the right knee closer to your chest. Slowly stretch the right leg closer to your shoulder loosening the hamstrings. Release the right leg down to a supine position.

Seated Middle Split

Samakonasana

Level: Advanced

Position: Sitting

Style: Stretch

Chakra: Root

Element: Earth

Anatomy Focus: Hips, Quadriceps

Begin in a seated position, Butterfly Pose. Straighten your spine. Lower both shoulders and engage your core. Inhale and exhale widening both legs to the corner of your mat. Tuck your lower back and place both hands firmly in front of you on the mat. Lower your chin to your chest and slowly roll forward supporting your upper body with both hands. Relax into the pose letting gravity assist with the fold. Inhale and exhale. Slowly roll up one vertebrae at a time back to a seated position.

Pigeon

Kapotasana

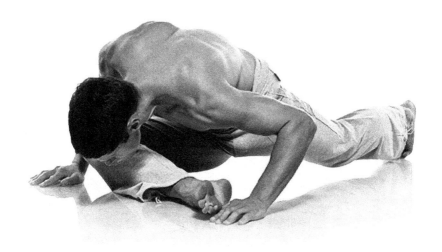

Level: Advanced

Position: Prone

Style: Stretch, Back-Bend

Chakra: Crown, Third Eye, Throat, Heart

Element: Thought, Light, Ether, Air

Anatomy Focus: Lower and Middle Back, Core, Hamstrings, Chest, Hips, Neck, Pelvic, Psoas, Quadriceps

Begin this pose in Table Top position. Bring your left knee to meet your left wrist. Inhale and lower your left hip to the floor, supporting your body with both hands on the mat. Keep your right leg straight behind your body, knee facing the floor. Lift your chest at this point for a deep stretch. Or, slowly lower your upper body over your left knee. Relax both elbows to the mat in front of you, palms down. Inhale and exhale. Push up through the palms of your hands and lift your chest of of your knees. Return to Child's pose.

Crane

Bakasana

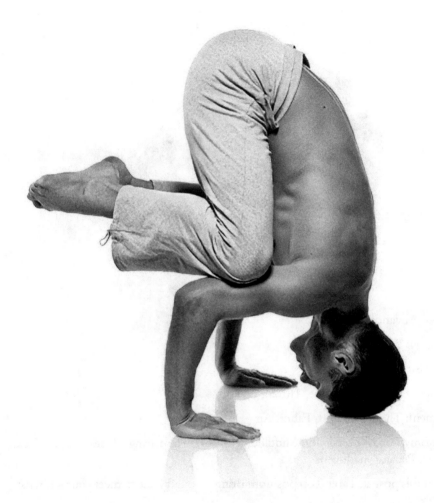

Level: Advanced

Position: Sitting

Style: Strength, Inversion, Balance

Chakra: Solar Plexus

Element: Fire

Anatomy Focus: Middle and Upper Back, Biceps and Triceps

Start this pose in a seated Garland pose. Inhale and exhale multiple times preparing for this pose. Place both palms on the floor engaging the triceps. Bring both knees to the chest and place them firmly in the armpit area. You will be on your tip toes at this point. Continue to allow a slight bend in both elbows. Take a few deep breaths. As you exhale, bend the torso forward lifted the buttocks in the air. Shift your weight onto your knees. Slowly lean forward pointing your forehead toward your mat. Allow both feet to lift off the mat while balancing your knees on top of your triceps. Inhale and exhale. Slowly roll back on to your feet and return to Garland Pose.

Headstand

Sirsasana

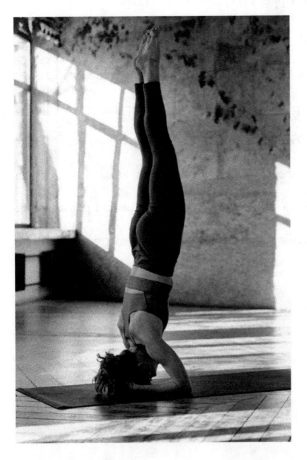

Level: Advanced

Position: Supine

Style: Inversion, Strength, Balance

Chakra: Crown, Third Eye, Throat

Element: Thought, Light, Ether

Anatomy Focus: Lower Back, Biceps and Triceps, Neck

Begin by kneeling on your mat. Rest your forearms on the mat shoulder width apart. Interlock your fingers and place the crown of your head on the mat. Cup the back of your head with your hands. After securing your head position, tuck both knees into your stomach. Inhale and exhale engaging your core and tightening the hip area. Begin to rest your weight onto your forearms and slowly lift one knee off the floor. Keep your heel close to your buttocks. Lift the opposite knee from the floor keeping both knees close to the lower body. Inhale and exhale and tightening the stomach muscles. Shift your weight off of your head and onto your elbows for balance. Slowly straighten both legs while engaging the core with every breath. Point your toes. Inhale and exhale. Gently lower one foot at a time back to a kneeling position. Slowly roll up to a final standing position.

Scorpion

Vrschikasana

Level: Advanced

Position: Prone

Style: Strength, Back-Bend, Inversion, Balance

Chakra: Crown, Third Eye, Throat

Element: Thought, Light, Ether

Anatomy Focus: Arms and Shoulders, Lower and Middle Back, Biceps and Triceps

Begin in Downward Dog. Lower both elbows down to the floor, resting both forearms on the mat. Follow the same steps as the Headstand pose to lift your feet into the air. Tuck both knees into your stomach. Inhale and exhale engaging your core and tightening the hip area. Begin to rest your weight onto your forearms and slowly lift one knee off the floor. Keep your heel close to your buttocks. Lift the opposite knee from the floor keeping both knees close to the lower body. Shift your weight onto your hands, forearms and elbows. Inhale and exhale. Slowly straighten both legs while engaging the core with every breath. Point your toes toward the sky. Inhale and exhale tightening the stomach muscles. Slowly begin to bend both knees. Point the toes toward the back of your head. Bend from the middle to upper back. Gently begin to lower one leg at a time back down to the mat. Relax back into Child's Pose.

PART III

Restorative Yoga Exercise #1

30 Minutes – 5 Poses

How to Set Up

You will need:

- 2 blocks/bricks
- 1 bolster
- 2 blankets
- 1 eye pillow
- 1 yoga mat
- 1 chair

Find a quiet and peaceful place to practice. Practicing in a dark or room with low light is best. Place your mat in an open and spacious area. Grab each prop and lay them next to your mat within arm's reach.

Pose #1 - Meditation

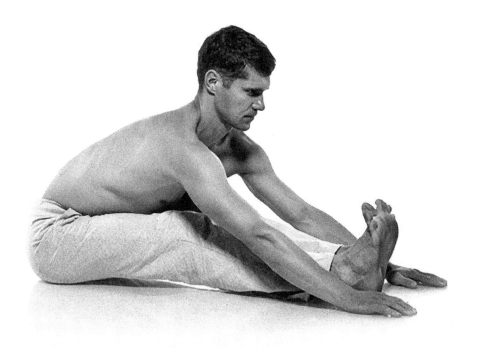

Begin in any comfortable seated position with one of the short edges of your mat against a wall. By placing your mat up against the wall at the beginning of each yoga practice, you will minimize having to move the mat multiple times.

Find your most comfortable position. You can sit on the floor, on a blanket, on your mat, in a chair, on a bolster, on a block, etc. Just make sure that you are in some form of a seated position. You're welcome to cross your legs, extend them straight in front of you, etc. Whatever feels the most comfortable and can help you to create a calm and relaxing space around your body.

(Refer to the "Hands to Heart" pose detailed in Chapter 1 "Yoga Poses.")

Meditation is a time to soften your body and bring awareness to your mind. Your meditation should be created specifically for you and no one else. It is your time to give your thoughts some much needed attention.

Close your eyes, begin to feel your breath. Touch your hands to your stomach to generate a deeper feel. Notice how your breath moves your body. Feel your body begin to create its own rhythm, flow and pace as you breath in through your nose and out through your mouth.

Take a few minutes to contine exhaling and inhaling, letting your heart rate settle into a solid pace. Feel free to quietly repeat a sound or to hum after each breath. Anything that provides a pace for you to follow as your continue to breath. These sounds are called "mantras" and can be quietly vocalized throughout your yoga session. If you are following the direction of an instructor, listen to their cues to release your mantra sounds.

Meditation can last as long as you would like it to last. If you have a specific amount of time allotted for your yoga routine (this routine is 30 minutes), try to give yourself about five minutes to sink into a state of meditation before beginning the following poses.

Pose #2 – Reclined with Bent Knees

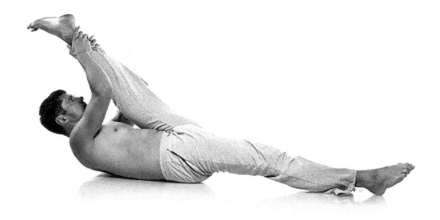

Use two blocks to support your bolster from moving backward. Or, if possible, place the shorter edge of your yoga mat up against an empty wall. Place the wide edge of the bolster up against that wall.

Begin in a seated position with your back facing the lower edge of your bolster. Place your lower back close enough to touch the bolster and bend your legs.

Slowly roll your lower body down onto the base of the inclined bolster. Inhale and exhale. Tuck your torso and fold your chin to your chest. These subtle movements will help to elongate your spine while rolling into the position on your incline. Gently roll your back down one vertebrae at a time onto the incline. Under each bent knee place a rolled blanket to support the knee.

Bring the soles of your feet together

Stack your blankets on each side to rest your elbows. Once you are comfortable, place a blanket over your body. Lean back onto the bolster using a blanket to support your head.

Place an eye pillow or scarf over your eyes and forehead to darken the space around you. Go ahead and rest your hands on your stomach. You can lace your fingers together or simply just place one hand on top of the other. Begin to feel you breath move your stomach up and down.

Restorative poses can last as long as you would like them to last. You are welcome to set a timer or simply just rest until you feel it is time to move on.

Pose #3 – Reclined with Legs Straight

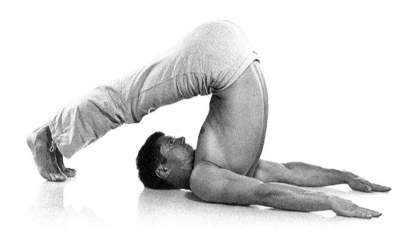

This pose begins very much like Pose #2. However, in this pose you will straighten your legs and prop either your block or your folded blanket under your knees or your legs. Your heels may feel pressure in this pose. Feel free to fold another blanket and prop it under the heels of both feet. If desired, cover yourself with your blanket and place your eye pillow or scarf in the same position, over your eyes and forehead. Sink into the restorative pose for as long as needed.

Pose #4 – Reclined with Legs on Chair

Props will change with this pose. Begin by removing everything from your mat. Let's start with a clean slate. Place your chair at the short end of your mat. Place two of the chair's legs on the mat to avoid slipping during this pose. If you have enough space, go ahead and put all four legs on the mat for optimal safety.

Place a folded blanket next to the chair as you lay down in supine position, on your back. The blanket should be long enough so that your shoulders are still on the mat when laying down. Make sure the blanket is wide enough for you to lay your entire body down on the mat. Drape the second blanket over the seat of the chair.

If you have extra blankets, fold them and place next to your mat, one for each elbow. Fold another blanket to use under your head as a cushion. If you do not have extra blankets, towels or small pillows will work as well.

Have two blankets close by before you put your feet up on the chair. Use one blanket to cover your feet and legs.

Begin in a seated position facing the open seat of your chair. Slowly roll down one vertebrae at a time with your back flat on your blanket. Bend your knees and place both calves flat on the seat of the chair. Grab the blankets for your elbows and head and place them accordingly. If the forehead tilts back, then place the blanket under the head and neck, but not the shoulders.

Place your eye pillow or scarf on your eyes and forehead.

Relax into the reclined chair pose.

To come out of the pose, slowly lower both legs back down to your mat. Move the chair as needed and transition to svasana, or corpse pose.

Pose #5 - Savasana

Relax in supine position on your mat. Let your arms float to the side of your hips, palms up. Extend your legs. Move the blankets under your knees if needed.

Adjust your head and neck by lifting your head and focusing down the middle of your body. Make sure you are evenly placed on the mat.

Gently lower the head and begin to let your entire body sink into the mat or blanket below. Follow the breathing methods in the meditation practice as mentioned in Pose #1.

Restorative Yoga Exercise #2

60 Minutes – 7 Poses

How to Setup:

You will need:

- 4 blocks/bricks

- 1 strap

- 1 bolster

- 1 blanket

- 1 yoga mat

Find a quiet and peaceful place to practice. Practicing in a dark or room with low light is best. Place your mat in an open and spacious area. Grab each prop and lay them next to your mat within arm's reach.

Pose #1

Meditation

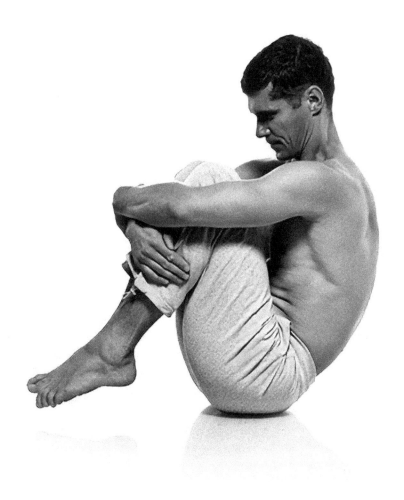

You will recognize a pattern of meditation for each Restorative exercise in this book. Beginning any yoga practice in a meditative state generates body awareness and mental focus.

To begin, place yourself in any comfortable seated position. Place one of the short edges of your mat against a wall.

Find your most comfortable position, on the floor, on a blanket, on your mat, in a chair, on a bolster, on a block, etc.

(Refer to the "Hands to Heart" pose detailed in Chapter 1 "Yoga Poses.")

Soften your body, relax each muscle and bring awareness to your mind. Listen to the sounds around your body. Can you hear other people breathing? Is the air conditioning or heat running? Are there shuffling feet outside the classroom doors? Do you hear birds or cars outside the window? Remember, this is your meditiation, your space, and your mind.

Close your eyes, begin to feel your breath. Feel your entire body move as you breath in through the nose and out through the mouth.

Pose #2

Upward Angle

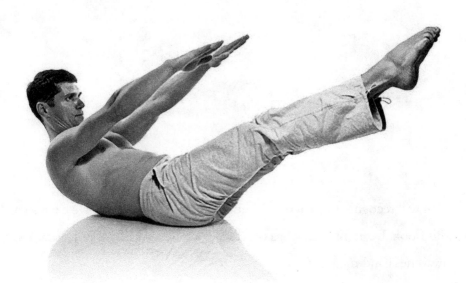

With your mat up against the empty wall, grab your strap. Make a loop in that strap. In a seated position, place your hip next to the wall.

Swing your legs up the wall and relax your torso on the floor. Place the loop in the strap around your calves. Make sure it is about midway up the calves to hold the legs.

If you have tight hamstrings (most of us do), move a few inches away from the wall. Do not strain the backs of your legs. They should be able to relax against the wall while in this pose.

Use the strap to stabilize the legs in the upward angle.

Allow your hamstrings to sink into the stretch for a few minutes. Release the straps, gently lower your legs.

Pose #3

Wide Angle

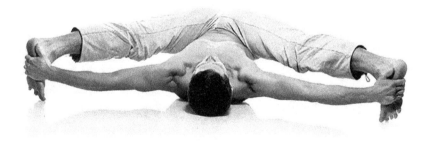

The wide angle pose is very much like Pose #2, the Upward Angle. There are a few changes.

Place two bricks on your mat and against the wall. Place your bolster against those bricks.

Sit your buttocks down on the bricks and let your lower back relax down the bolster.

Recline back on the bolster supporting your neck with your hands as needed. Roll a blanket and place it under your neck for support.

Place both of the legs straight up and flat against the wall.

Let your arms fall wide off of your mat, palms up.

Take the legs wide. Use a strap as needed. Loop the strap around one calf and hold.

Pose #4

Reclined Angle

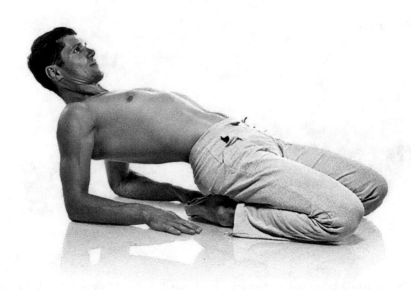

Leaving your mat in the same position, place two bricks together perpendicular to the wall. Place two more bricks within arm's reach.

Begin seated in from of the wall and place the soles of your feet evenly together. Keep your torso flat on your mat. Support your back with your bolster or with a folded blanket as needed.

Place one brick under your left hip and the last brick underneath your right hip. Gently lower both knees out to the side.

Gently allow the knees fall to the each side.

Tuck your shoulder blades and relax your neck. Lay both arms out wide. Use blanket props as needed for the neck and hands.

Stay in this pose for about five minutes.

To come out of the pose, bring your hands close to your side and close the knees. Roll to one side and press up to a seated position.

Pose #5

Front Side Body Stretch

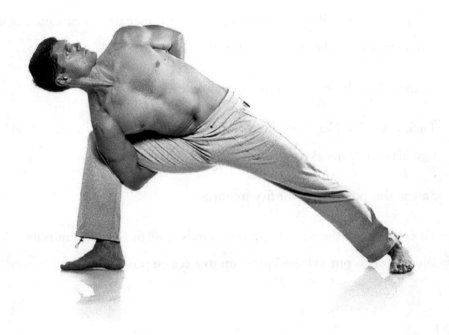

Let's grab 3-4 bricks for this one. This is an intense side stretch and will need a good amount of support for safety.

Place the bricks in a line on the center of the mat, 1 at each height, in order.

Sit in front of the first brick, then hold that brick in one hand. Bend your knees.

Begin to recline backwards over the middle brick. Continue to lay back until the shoulders reach the end of that middle brick. Allow the head to rest down onto the third brick in the row.

Put pressure on the soles of both feet. Next, place the brick that is in your hand under your sacrum and lower body area.

Continue to extend your legs in front of your body, If you are next to a wall, press your feet in to the wall keeping the heels on the floor. If you would like, place a fourth brick underneath both calves. If you do not have a fourth brick, you can use a folded blanket or a small pillow.

Rest in this position.

To come out of the pose, gently press into the soles of your feet, bend your knees and roll into a seated position.

Pose #6

Bridge Pose on Blocks

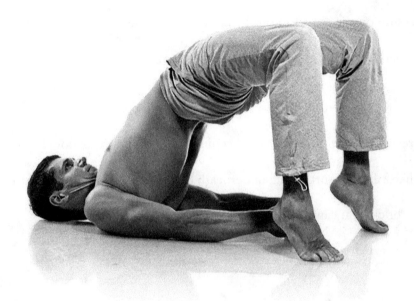

Let's grab four blocks and your blanket for this pose. Take the first two

blocks and place them at a medium height in the middle of your mat. Place

the third and fourths blocks at a lower height next to the first two.

Place the blanket under your lower back for sacrum support. You may

want to avoid placing a blanket under your neck for this pose since you

will be in an inverted position.

Next, grab the third brick and place it in your hand. Sit your buttocks in the place of the third block. Face the wall, bend your knees and place the soles of your feet flat on the floor.

Slowly lay back on the last brick. Place the bottom edge of your shoulder blades on the brick. Let the upper shoulders lay completely on the mat.

Now, you will still have that third brick in your hand. Place it under your sacrum and lower back area for optimatl support. Press through the soles of your feet and allow your upper body to rest gently on your shoulders.

Inhale and exhale while resting in this postion for a few minutes.

Pose #7 - Savasana

We will end each exercise with Savasana. It is important to transition your mind and body out of any exercise through some form of meditation or relaxation.

Let's mimic Pose #5 from Exercise #1. Feel free to modify depending on what works for you. Savasana may change for you with each routine. That is perfectly alright. Each day is different. Therefore, let your yoga practice evolve each day as well.

Relax in supine position on your mat. Let your arms float to the side of your hips, palms up. Extend your legs. Move the blankets under your knees if needed.

Adjust your head and neck by lifting your head and focusing down the middle of your body. Make sure you are evenly placed on the mat.

Gently lower the head and let your entire body sink into the mat or blanket below.

Follow the breathing methods in the meditation practice as mentioned in Part 2 of this book as well as in Pose #1 of this exercise.

Restorative Yoga

Exercise #3

75 Minutes – 6 Poses

How to Setup

You will need:

- 1 yoga mat
- 1 strap or belt
- 1 bolster

Find a quiet and peaceful place to practice. Practicing in a dark or room with low light is best. Place your mat in an open and spacious area. Grab each prop and lay them next to your mat within arm's reach.

Pose #1

Meditation

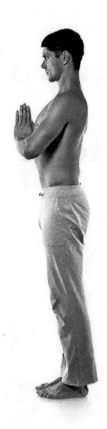

Once again, we begin in meditation. Find the most comfortable position for your body - on the floor, on a blanket, on your mat, in a chair, on a bolster, on a block, etc.

(Refer to the "Hands to Heart" pose detailed in Chapter 1 "Yoga Poses.")

Cross your legs, extend the legs, widen the legs. It's up to you. Let your hands drift softly by your side or on to the tops of your knees. You can place your hands, palms up, or palms down. As always, be comfortable.

Close your eyes, begin to feel your breath. Touch your hands to your stomach to generate a deeper feel for how your breath moves your body. Feel your body begin to create its own rhythm, flow and pace yourself as you breath in through your nose and out through your mouth.

The simple act of inhaling and exhaling brings awareness to your mind and oxygen to your muscles.

Pose #2

Captured Butterfly

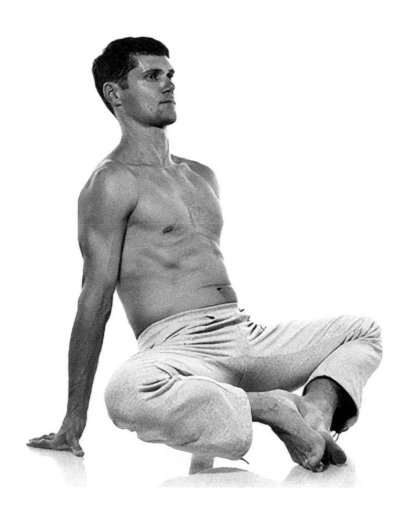

Ok, let's open up those hips! Place your bolster behind you lengthwise. Situate the bolster so that it is parallel to the long edge of your yoga mat. In a seated position, place your lower backside against that long edge of the bolster.

Grab your strap and make a wide loop at one end. Hold the tail end of your strap. Begin by placing the loop over your head and move it all the way down to your pelvic area.

Still in your seated position, bend both knees and touch the soles of both feet. Open both knees out wide, letting gravity complete the stretch. Take two of your blankets, fold them into rectangles and lay them under your knees as needed.

Swing the loop of your strap around both feet. Let it land in the middle of the sole of each foot.

Tighten your strap, and allow it to hold your legs securely in this position.

Roll down on your back onto your bolster. Remember to keep your chin pointed toward your chest and to tuck your torso as you roll down. This will lengthen your spine as you relax into the position. You can place both arms down by your side, out wide, or place them above your head. Fold a blanket and put it underneath your head or neck simply for comfort. The support will keep your neck from tilting back.

Let all of your muscles sink into this position and relax for a few minutes.

While in each position, you can return to your meditative breathing. Also, take some time to let your eyes sink back into your eye sockets to soften the face muscles.

Repeat your "ohm" sounds if desired.

Let's go ahead and come out of this pose. Gently press into your forearms to slowly lift yourself back up to a seated position.

Release the strap around your feet, lean forward and bend your knees. Slowly roll up to a seated position.

Pose #3

Mermaid

For this pose, we will need our bolster and some blankets.

Stay in your seated position, bend both knees and put both feet flat on the floor. Each foot should be about hip-distance apart.

Slowly lower both knees toward the right, and pivot your torso slightly in the same direction.

Lower the right side of your body toward the bolster. Rest on your right shoulder.

Rest your head and neck down onto your hands or your bolster below. Fold a blanket and prop your head if needed.

Close your eyes and let gravity do the rest. Let each muscle sink into your mat and your bolster. It may help to think of each muscle from your head to your toes. Begin by letting your toes loosen, then your feet, then legs, torso, chest, all the way to your forehead muscles.

After relaxing into this position, slowly press up with your hands.

Twisted positions may sometimes cause a tingling in our limbs. If this begins to happen, make sure to reposition your arms or legs to redirect the circulation.

Repeat these steps on the left side.

Pose #4

Constructive Rest Pose

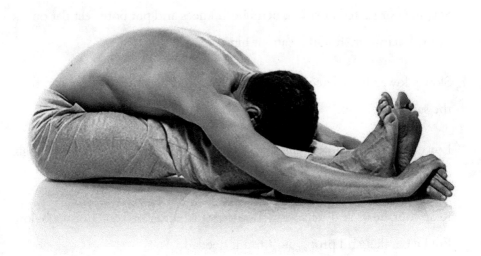

Alright, let's move our bolster out of the way for this pose. However, let's keep our strap with the loop. We will need that prop.

Grab that strap and loop it around your legs. Slide it up to your thighs, just above both knees.

Place both feet flat on the floor. Go ahead and let them rest wide, about as wide as your mat.

Tighten the strap around your legs for control. Obviously, do not tighten the strap too much. We don't want to cut off any blood circulation.

Now that your legs are in the proper position, slowly roll down, one vertebrae at a time onto your back.

Cross your right arm under your left arm, like you are giving yourself a full body hug. Relax both shoulders. This movement tends to cause us to tense our shoulders and neck areas. Lower those shoulders away from the ears.

Relax your hands and allow the wrists and forearms to hang loosely.

After a few minutes, switch arms positions.

Sink deeper into the stretch for a few more minutes. Untwist both arms and push back up to your seated position.

Pose #5

Legs Up the Wall

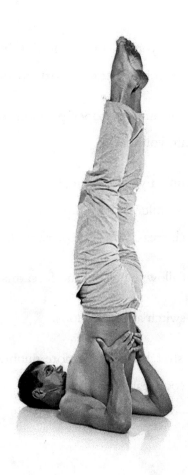

Ok, let's make our way to the wall. Make sure it's an empty wall so that nothing can fall and cause injury.

Sit facing the wall on your mat. Walk both feet up the wall. Scoot yourself closer to the wall. You can touch your lower body to the wall or slide back a few inches. Whatever is most comfortable.

Relax the knees and let your arms lay beside your hips.

If you would like to grab a bolster, place it underneath your body for support. If you decide to use the bolster, make sure that your entire upper body is horizontal. Your back should be completely supported by the bolster.

Slide your buttocks slightly off the bolster so that you are closer to the wall.

Close your eyes and continue to inhale and exhale. Feel the movement of your stomach muscles as they tighten and release.

To come out of the pose, slowly bend your kness and press your feet into the wall. Slide your body away from the wall and return to an upright position.

Pose #6 - Savasana

Now, for our favorite pose!

If needed, refer to Pose #5 from Exercise #1. Remember to modify Savasana depending on what works for you.

Relax in supine position on your mat. Let your arms float to the side of your hips, palms up. Extend your legs. Move the blankets under your knees if needed.

Adjust your head and neck by lifting your head and focusing down the middle of your body. Make sure you are evenly placed on the mat.

Gently lower the head and begin to let your entire body sink into the mat or blanket below. Soften the weight of your body and relax the muscles in your face.

Follow the breathing methods in "Meditation" as mentioned in Pose #1.

Close your eyes. Let both arms relax by your sides. Turn the palms up toward the sky. Let your body sink into this pose.

Inhale and exhale.

Enjoy this Savasana for about 5-10 minutes.

Restorative Yoga

Exercise #4

90 Minutes – 13 Poses – 3 Setup Options

How to Setup

You will need:

- 2 blocks
- 2 bolsters
- 2 blankets
- 1 yoga mat

Find a quiet and peaceful place to practice. Practicing in a dark or room with low light is best. Place your mat in an open and spacious area. Grab each prop and lay them next to your mat within arm's reach.

Situate your bolster slanting up on the edge of your mat. You are welcome to place your bolster anywhere on your mat.

Here are three exercises with different variations for props. Props may be manufactured differently. Some bolsters may be more firm than others. And, blocks and bricks may not be the exact same size. Modify poses based on how the props work with your unique physique. And, most importantly, make sure that you are comfortable.

Setup #1 With a Bolster

With a firm bolster, place a block on its side horizontally toward the edge of your mat. Lay one of the short ends of your bolster on it. This will put the highest edge of your bolster toward the edge of your mat. If you have a bolster that is softer, fold your blanket on top of the block for additional support. You can use this modification for each of the poses below.

Setup #2 – Without a Bolster

This pose can be done without a bolster. We will use a blanket for modification. So, if you don't have a bolster, fold two blankets into rectangles. Lay the blankets on top of one another. This will create a makeshift bolster. Depending on your height, add blankets as needed. It is very important to remember to modify as needed based on your body size. Place two blocks underneath the blankets if needed. This will prop each blanket up for more support. Place one block at the very back of your mat. Place a second block directly in front of the first block.

Lay each of the blankets over the blocks. The blankets will tilt upwards toward the back of the mat.

Setup #3

Place the first bolster horizontally toward the edge of your mat. Place the second bolster lengthwise along the mat. Rest the short end of that bolster on the first bolster. This will create a slanted edge and inclines the bolster.

Once you've inclined your bolster, you're ready to make yourself comfortable in the following poses.

Each of these incline setups can be used in your everyday life. You can set up on your bed while you read, on your couch while watching TV or just on the floor if you need a lower back stretch.

Pose #1 - Meditation

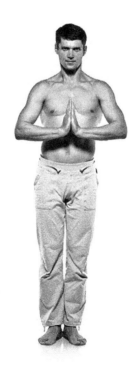

Begin in any comfortable seated position with one of the short edges of your mat against a wall. By placing your mat up against the wall at the beginning of each yoga practice, you will minimize having to move the mat multiple times.

Find your most comfortable position. You can sit on the floor, on a blanket, on your mat, in a chair, on a bolster, on a block, etc. Just make sure that you are in some form of a seated position.

(Refer to the "Hands to Heart" pose detailed in Chapter 1 "Yoga Poses.")

You are welcome to cross your legs, extend them straight out in front of you, etc. Whatever feels the most comfortable and can help you to create a calm space around your body.

Meditation is a time for you to soften your body and bring awareness to your mind. Your meditation should be created specifically for you and no one else.

Close your eyes, begin to feel your breath. Touch your hands to your stomach to generate a deeper feel for how your breath moves your body. Feel your body begin to create its own rhythm and flow as your breath in through your nose and out through your mouth.

Pose #2 - Reclining Tree Pose

In a seated position on your mat, extend your legs in front of you. Slowly roll your lower body down onto the base of the bolster. Inhale and exhale sure this motion. Tuck your torso and fold your chin to your chest. These subtle movements will help to elongate your spine while rolling into the position on your incline.

Gently roll your back one vertebrae at a time onto the incline. Support your lower body by placing your hands, palms down, on the mat beside your hips. Or, for a stronger core, straighten both arms in front of you as you lower your upper body. Rest your arms down to your mat.

After positioning yourself in an supine position on your incline, continue inhaling and exhaling. Bend your right knee. Slowly let it fall to the side of your body on your mat. Bring your right foot inward and let the sole of that foot touch your thigh. Lay both arms out to the side of your body, palms facing up. After a few minutes here, repeat on the left side.

If you need more props:

Place a blanket under your head if your neck is uncomfortable. If your chin is facing the ceiling, use the blanket for support. Fold the blanket as many times as necessary. Your neck should feel relaxed during this pose. Do not add the blanket if your neck is not strained in this position. Sometimes added support can force the neck forward, causing an awkward placement.

If your hips, thighs or any part of your lower body begin to hurt or feel pressure during this pose, place a blanket or bolster under your back or knees. The prop should alleviate any pressure in those areas. Sometimes your hands or wrists may not lay completely on the mat or floor. If this is an issue, place a blanket under both hands or wrists for more support. They should not feel strained during this pose. Your entire body should feel supported during this pose. The added support allows gravity to work and your body to sink into a completely relaxed state.

Pose #3 - Reclined Angle Pose

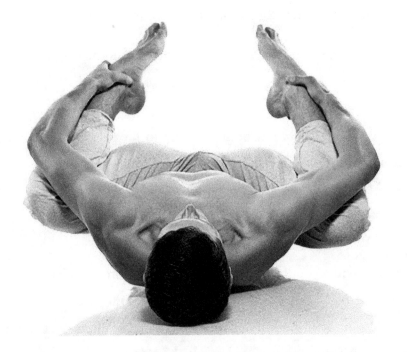

In seated position, recline down on your back onto your bolster. You will be in an inclined supine position again. Roll down slowly. Remember to tuck your torso and place your chin on your chest to elongate your spine while slowly rolling down onto your inclined bolster. Bend both of your knees and lower them onto your mat. Bring your feet together, soles touching. Your feet can be as close to your body or as far away from your body as needed. Position them so that your sacrum area feels relaxed. Lie in this position for several minutes.

If you need more props:

Once again, add a folded blanket under your head if your neck is strained. Use the blankets, bolster, or blocks under your knees or lower body. Sometimes when we position our knees outward, our inner thighs and hips will feel extra tension. Placing these support props under the tense areas allow the muscle to loosen and relax properly. Place blankets under the your hands and wrists again if needed.

Straps can also come in handy during this pose. Make a loop with the strap, slip it over your head, place it near your sacrum. Pull it through from the inside of your thighs, and loop it around your feet. Let the strap tighten slightly for a gentle hug and a supported deeper stretch. Utlizing the strap will tilt your pelvis slightly and keep your feet together.

Pose #4 - Reclined Twist

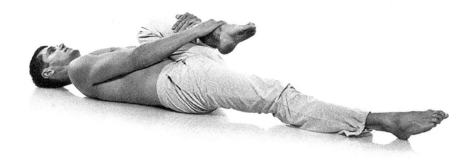

In a seated position on your mat, extend your legs in front of you. Roll your lower body down onto the base of the inclined bolster. Tuck your torso and fold your chin to your chest. Remember to continue inhaling and exhaling as your make your way down to your inclined position.

Once you are in a comfortable position on your back against your incline, bend your knees and place the soles of your feet on the mat. Make sure to keep the knees about hip-width apart. Touching both knees together, move your bent legs slowly from side to side. You don't need to touch the ground each time. Gently sway the legs left to right. After a few movements, let both legs fall to one side. Continue the same motion, and then let the knees fall to the opposite side. Repeat as desired.

If you need more props:

Add a folded blanket under your head if your neck is strained. Use the blankets, bolster, or blocks under your knees or lower body. Blankets or bolsters can be used on either side of the mat to support your knees as you drop them to the side. A blanket can also be placed in between your thighs to cushion the weight of the top leg when relaxing them to either side. Position the blanket between the knees as well if you begin to feel pressure on your joint area. Add your folded blankets for your arms, hands and wrists as needed.

Pose #5 - Supported Fish

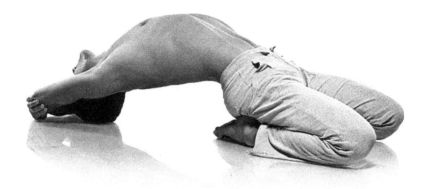

In a seated position on your mat, extend your legs in front of you. Much like the Tree pose, slowly roll your lower body down onto the base of your incline. Inhale and exhale during this motion. Tuck your torso and fold your chin to your chest. Roll back onto your incline. Extend your legs in front of your body on your mat. Relax into this position.

If you need more props:

If your neck is uncomfortable, place a blanket under your head. Roll one of your blankets and place it under your knees. This tilts and supports your lower back as you extend your legs into the stretch. Loop a strap around your ankles to keep your feet together during the pose. Place blankets under your hands, wrists and elbows as needed.

Pose #6 - Reclined Side Bend

From a reclining position on your bolster with your legs straight out in front of you, move your right foot a few inches to the right. Cross your left ankle over your right ankle. Keep your arms next to your body. You could also place your hands above or behind your head for part or all of your time in this pose.

You can also arch your upper body if your back allows the stretch. After a few minutes here, repeat on the left side.

If you need more props:

Fold a blanket or two and place it under your head for support. Blankets can also be placed under your arms and hands for proper alignment and comfort.

Pose #7 - Locust

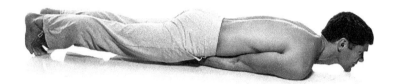

Begin in a seated position. Turn your body over and lift up on all fours – Table Top pose. Situate the bottom of your bolster next to both knees. Slowly lower your stomach to the floor. Move your shins and feet up the incline of the bolster. Stack your hands to make a pillow for your forehead. You can also fold multiple blankets as a cushion for your forehead as well.

This is a restorative back bend post. If you would like a deeper back bend, move your pelvis closer to the bolster. That way, your thighs, knees and shins will be elevated. Be very careful if you have any type of back injury. A deeper bend may not be the best option.

As you inhale and exhale, draw your stomach muscles away from the mat for a deeper stretch.

If you need more props:

You may need to place a blanket under your front hip bones for added comfort. Also, loop your strap around your ankles to hold both feet in place.

Sometimes stretching your arms behind your back releases tension in the lower back. If you would like to place your arms behind your back, place a folded blanket under your forehead. Make sure you have room to continue breathing through your nose and mouth. Place a block under the front of each shoulder for a slight lift if desired.

Pose #8 - Prone Twist

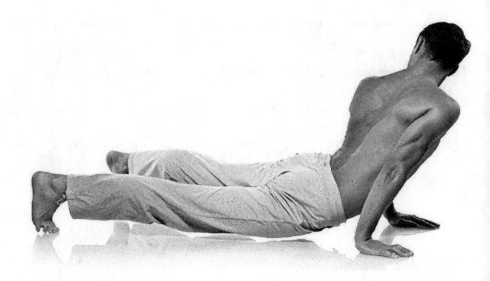

Sitting up, place your left hip against the base of the bolster. Bend both knees and point them to the left. Turn your torso toward the bolster and place both hands on the mat beside that bolster. Slowly lower your torso down. Let your chest rest softly on the incline of the bolster.

Wrap your arms around the bolster or let both arms relax beside the bolster. Lay the side of your face down onto the bolster. Either side is fine. Turn your face in the opposite direction of your knees for a deeper side stretch.

Relax into this position for a few minutes. Repeat the twist on the opposite side. If at any time you begin to feel numbness or a tingling anywhere in the body during a twist post, slowly come out of the pose. This will restore proper circulation.

If you need more props:

Fold a blanket and place it between your knees. You can also use a blanket as a cushion between your outer knee and the floor/mat.

Pose #9 - Child's Pose

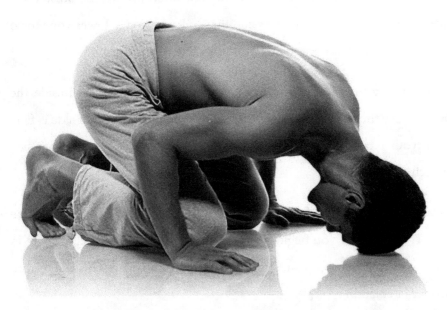

Let's stretch that lower back. Begin in table top pose – on all fours. Sit back onto your heels. Separate your knees so that you are almost straddling the lower part of the bolster. Slowly fold forward and lower your chest down to the top of the bolster. Keep your buttocks on top of your heels.

Let the shoulders relax away from your ears. Hug the bolster or slide your arms behind you, palms up.

Lay your head to one side. Relax the muscles. Lift your head and slowly turn it in the opposite direction. Continue to inhale and exhale. Feel your chest move your upper body as you breath in and out.

If you need more props:

As you lay forward, the weight of your body may create some pressure on your knees. Add a folded blanket behind the knees.

Pose #10 - Forward Fold – Wide Legs

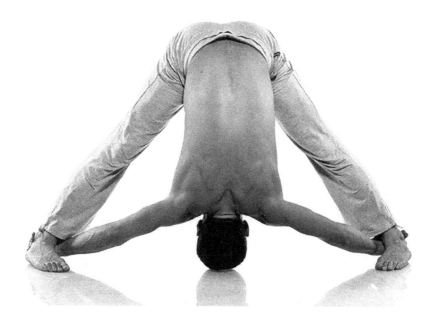

In a seated upright position, face the bolster. Widen the legs and straddle the lower part of your bolster. Your legs should be straight in this postion. Fold forward and lay your chest on top of the bolster. Stack your hands underneath your head or place a blanket as a cushion. Rest your forearms and hands on the floor. Relax your head to one side. Halfway through the pose, turn your face in the opposite direction.

If you need more props:

This forward fold may be more comfortable by adding a few folded blankets underneath your lower body. You can also fold forward in this pose with bent knees. Add a block under each knee for support if you choose this option.

Your heels may begin to feel some pressure if you have chosen to straighten both legs. If so, add folded blankets under both heels to soften the weight. Also, if your hands are uncomfortable underneath your head, use a blanket or small pillow instead.

This pose can also be done without the bolster. Sometimes the bolster can cause the hamstrings to feel strained. Move the bolster and set it up vertically. With the bolster in this position, you can rest your forehead. Set your head against the top of the bolster as you fold forward. This will relieve the tight hamstrings as well.

Pose #11 - One Leg Prop

Let's first place the bolster at the end of our mat, near our feet. Begin this pose lying down on your back. Place your head at the short edge of your mat. Move slightly to the left side of your mat. Lie down on your back with your head at the front of your mat. Place your right leg on the bolster and your left leg on the mat.

Let both arms fall to your side, palms facing up. You are also welcome to lay your hands on your stomach. Rest in this pose for a few minutes. Allow your lower back and sacrum area to sink into your mat. Remember to continue to breathe with each movement.

If you need more props:

Use a folded blanket for your neck. Support your forearms, wrists and hands with a few extra blankets as well.

Another great option: place two blocks on either side of your head. These will keep your head from turning. The placement of the blocks may also drown out distracting sounds.

Pose #12 - Cow Face

Begin in a supine position on your mat. Lay flat on your back and prop both legs on the bolster. Cross your right leg over your left leg and bend both knees. Bring your feet to the floor on either side of the bolster.

Once again, rest your hands on your stomach or alongside your body. Rest in this position for a few minutes. Repeat on the opposite side.

Remember to come out of these twisted positions if you ever begin to feel numbness or tingling in any part of the body to restore circulation.

If you need more props:

Your neck may feel strained in this position. Place a small pillow under your head for added support. You can also grab your bolster or a blanket and fold it lengthwise on your torso for comfort.

Pose #13 - Legs Up/Savasana

For the final pose, lie down on your back, bringing both legs onto the bolster. The legs should be reaching "up" the bolster incline.

Relax in supine position. Let your arms float to the side of your hips, palms up. You can also rest your hands on your stomach if that feels more comfortable. Extend your legs. Move the blankets under your knees if needed.

Adjust your head and neck by lifting your head and focusing down the middle of your body. Make sure you are evenly placed on the mat.

Gently lower the head and begin to let your entire body sink into the mat or blanket below.

Let your upper, middle and lower back "melt" into the mat. Drop both shoulders. Release the fingers and the toes. Loosen the muscles in your arms and legs. Relax the eyes back into your eye sockets. Bring awareness to your tongue. Allow the muscles in your tongue to release, and let your lips open slightly.

Follow a slow and repetitive breathing pattern. Feel your stomach move up and down with each breath.

Become aware of your thoughts. With your eyes closed, you may begin to see a certain color. Let your mind drift toward that color as your thoughts drift to the back of your mind.

Inhale and exhale. Lay back and let your body finally relax into the next few minutes of silence, calmness and serenity.

Rest in this position for as long as you please.

As you begin to come out of this pose, let your eyes slowly flutter open. Take a deep breath in through your nose and exhale through the mouth. Roll to one side, press up through the palms of your hands and return your body to a "Hands to Heart" seated position.

Namaste

CPSIA information can be obtained
at www.ICGtesting.com
Printed in the USA
LVHW082234021020
667642LV00004B/97